Report of the Regional Director
on the work of WHO in the European
Region in 2010–2011

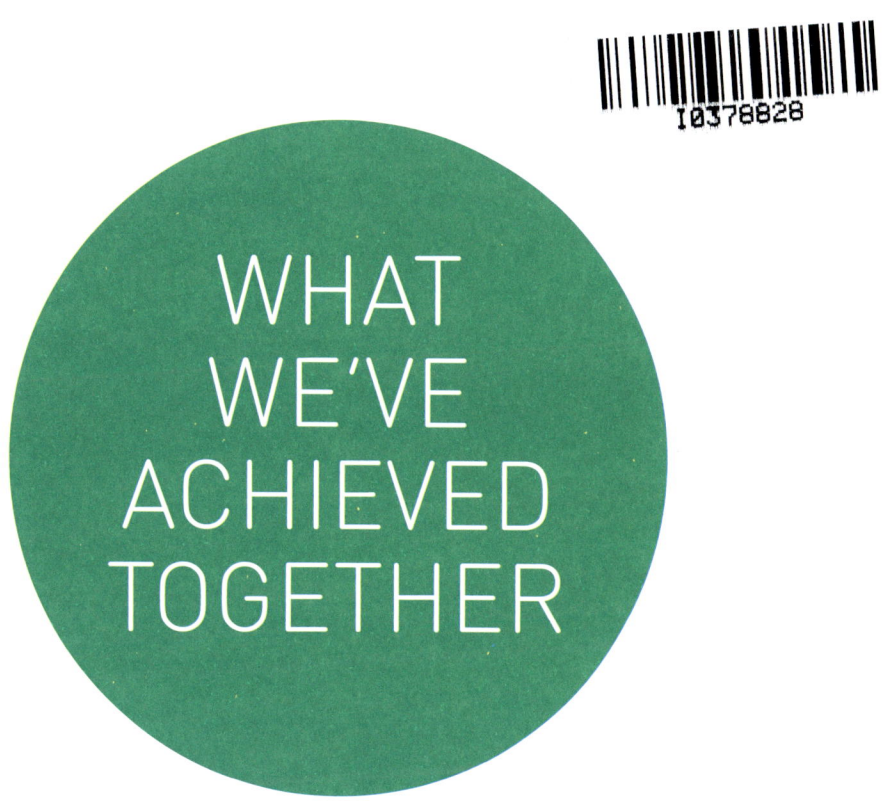

The World Health Organization was established in 1948 as the specialized agency of the United Nations serving as the directing and coordinating authority for international health matters and public health. One of WHO's constitutional functions is to provide objective and reliable information and advice in the field of human health. It fulfils this responsibility in part through its publications programmes, seeking to help countries make policies that benefit public health and address their most pressing public health concerns.

The WHO Regional Office for Europe is one of six regional offices throughout the world, each with its own programme geared to the particular health problems of the countries it serves. The European Region embraces nearly 900 million people living in an area stretching from the Arctic Ocean in the north and the Mediterranean Sea in the south and from the Atlantic Ocean in the west to the Pacific Ocean in the east. The European programme of WHO supports all countries in the Region in developing and sustaining their own health policies, systems and programmes; preventing and overcoming threats to health; preparing for future health challenges; and advocating and implementing public health activities.

To ensure the widest possible availability of authoritative information and guidance on health matters, WHO secures broad international distribution of its publications and encourages their translation and adaptation. By helping to promote and protect health and prevent and control disease, WHO's books contribute to achieving the Organization's principal objective – the attainment by all people of the highest possible level of health.

Report of the Regional Director on the work of WHO in the European Region in 2010–2011

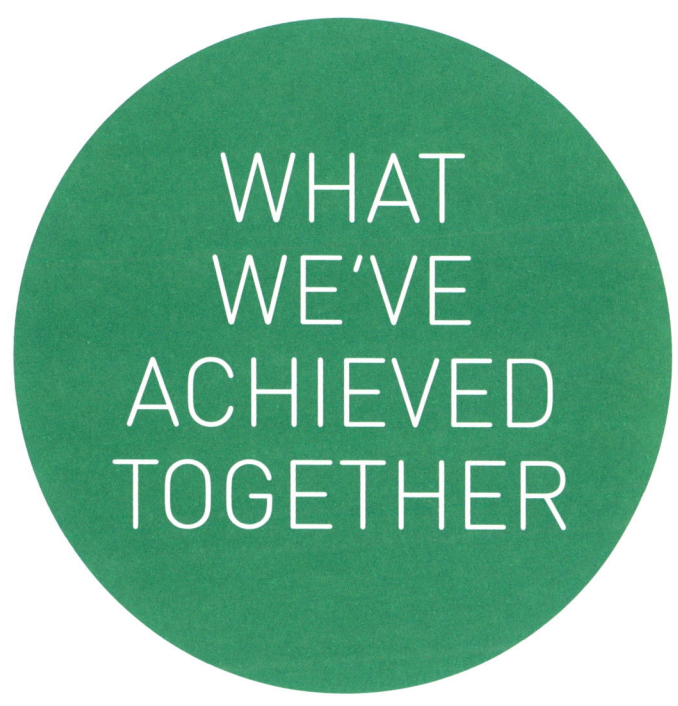

WHAT WE'VE ACHIEVED TOGETHER

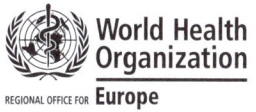

WHO Library Cataloguing-in-Publication Data

What we've achieved together : report of the Regional Director on the work of WHO in the European Region in 2010–2011.

1.Regional health planning. 2.World Health Organization. 3.Europe I.World Health Organization. Regional Office for Europe.

ISBN 978 92 890 1425 0 (print)   (NLM classification: WA 540)
ISBN 978 92 890 1426 7 (e-book)

ISBN 978 92 890 1425 0

Address requests about publications of the WHO Regional Office for Europe to:

    Publications
    WHO Regional Office for Europe
    Scherfigsvej 8
    DK-2100 Copenhagen Ø, Denmark

Alternatively, complete an online request form for documentation, health information, or for permission to quote or translate, on the Regional Office web site (http://www.euro.who.int/pubrequest).

© **World Health Organization 2012**

All rights reserved. The Regional Office for Europe of the World Health Organization welcomes requests for permission to reproduce or translate its publications, in part or in full.

The designations employed and the presentation of the material in this publication do not imply the expression of any opinion whatsoever on the part of the World Health Organization concerning the legal status of any country, territory, city or area or of its authorities, or concerning the delimitation of its frontiers or boundaries. Dotted lines on maps represent approximate border lines for which there may not yet be full agreement.

The mention of specific companies or of certain manufacturers' products does not imply that they are endorsed or recommended by the World Health Organization in preference to others of a similar nature that are not mentioned. Errors and omissions excepted, the names of proprietary products are distinguished by initial capital letters.

All reasonable precautions have been taken by the World Health Organization to verify the information contained in this publication. However, the published material is being distributed without warranty of any kind, either express or implied. The responsibility for the interpretation and use of the material lies with the reader. In no event shall the World Health Organization be liable for damages arising from its use. The views expressed by authors, editors, or expert groups do not necessarily represent the decisions or the stated policy of the World Health Organization.

CONTENTS

What we've achieved together 1
The vision: adoption and content 2
Progress towards the milestones
in 2010–2011 3
About this report 5

Overarching priorities 6
New European health policy: Health 2020 6
Essential support: corporate functions 8

Communicable diseases 17
HIV/AIDS 17
Tuberculosis 18
Malaria 19
Vaccine-preventable diseases
and immunization 19
Influenza 22
Antimicrobial resistance 23

Noncommunicable diseases 25
European action plan shaped
in a global context 25
Alcohol 26
Tobacco control 27
Nutrition 27
Mental health 28
Injuries 29
Patient, citizen and community
empowerment 30
Support to country-based activities
on individual diseases 30

**Health promotion throughout
the life-course** 31
Maternal and perinatal health 31
Childhood and adolescence 31

Sexual and reproductive health 32
Active and healthy ageing 33
MDGs 33
Ottawa Charter for Health Promotion 34

Strengthening of health systems 35
Strengthening of health systems 35
Supporting universal coverage and minimizing
the effects of the financial crisis 36
Action plan to strengthen public health 37
Support to health personnel 37
Patient empowerment 38
Information 38

Environment and health 39
Next steps in the European environment
and health process 39
Environmental determinants of health 40
Chernobyl commemoration 41

Preparedness, surveillance and response 42
IHR implementation and compliance 42
Preparedness 42
Alert and response 43

**Evidence and information as basis
for policy-making** 45
Integrated health-information system
and strategy for Europe 45
Tools 46
Publishing 46

References 47

**Annex. Implementation of the
programme budget for 2010–2011** 59

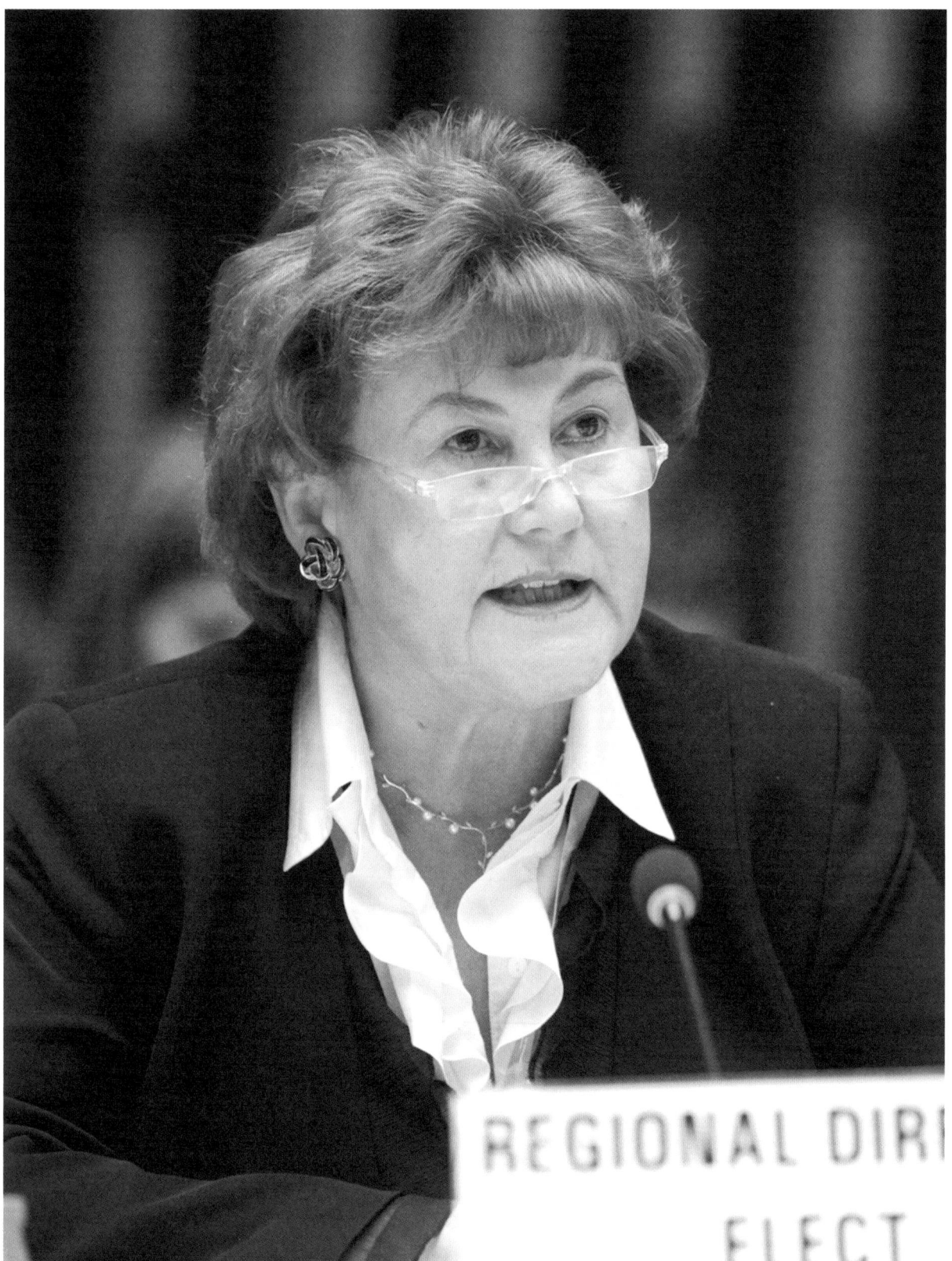

WHAT WE'VE ACHIEVED TOGETHER

Zsuzsanna Jakab

I took office as WHO Regional Director for Europe on 1 February 2010, with a vision for improving health in Europe by adapting the WHO Regional Office for Europe and its work to better support the 53 diverse Member States in the European Region. This vision was based on recognition of two essential facts. First, the WHO Regional Office for Europe could not continue doing business as usual, if it was to face the changes and challenges in the European Region and worldwide. These included: gaps in health and health-system development within and between countries, epidemiological changes such as the epidemic of noncommunicable diseases in Europe, the challenges of the financial crisis, the opportunities offered by the value given to health as a driver of growth, the strength of the scientific knowledge base and developments in information technology.

Second, developing, adopting, pursuing and ultimately achieving the vision required not "I", but "we". WHO in the European Region comprises both the Member States and the Secretariat in the Regional Office, which in turn is part of one WHO worldwide. More, in working for health, the meaning of "we" extends beyond WHO to all its partners in the Region.

This is my first report as Regional Director; it shows how we, in this broadest sense, started work and are well on the way to realizing the vision: setting Europe's priorities in 2010 and beginning to tackle its most urgent health issues in 2011, thus laying the foundation for the future.

The vision: adoption and content

In 2010, the Regional Office boldly proposed an ambitious vision for health development in Europe (1), and the WHO Regional Committee for Europe adopted it (2), committing both the Regional Office and Member States to realizing it over the following five years and agreeing on a road map with specific milestones on the way.

The elements of the vision and the external challenges faced had implications for the way that WHO engages in the European Region. All required discussion and agreement with the Regional Committee after appropriate preparatory work in its Standing Committee (SCRC). Checking on progress towards the milestones would ensure regular feedback to, input from and discussion with the Region's governing bodies and Member States. The progress made towards these milestones shows that WHO in the European Region is well on the way to realizing its vision. In 2010–2011, it followed the road map agreed, and delivered many of the items specified, as well as taking on an additional challenge: contributing to WHO reform (3,4). These achievements were made while the Regional Office dealt with several urgent and substantial emergencies, not least the flooding of the office in Copenhagen, Denmark in summer 2010 and 2011.

Goals and priorities

The overall objective is, within five years, to make the WHO Regional Office for Europe a stronger evidence-based centre of health policy and public health excellence, relevant to the whole Region,

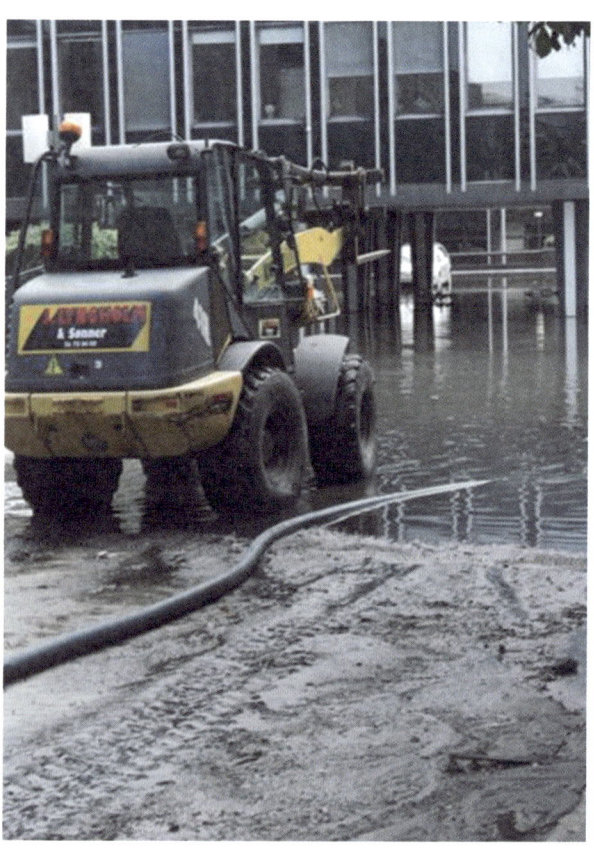
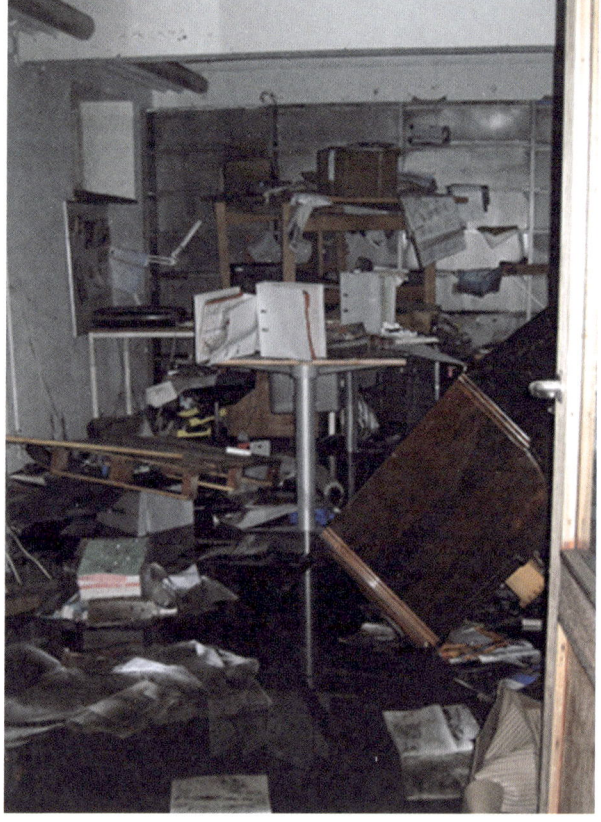

and with highly professional and motivated staff delivering high-quality technical programmes. It will have stronger, well-established and strategic partnerships with European and global actors and be fully engaged with them in joint action for better and more equal health in Europe and the world. Achieving this objective requires not only a clear mandate from WHO's governing bodies and the Member States but also their full support, continued guidance and active participation. With this in mind, the milestones set were linked to sessions of the Regional Committee.

To realize this vision, the Regional Office worked intensively on seven strategic priorities in 2010–2011:

1. developing a European health policy as a coherent policy framework that addresses all the challenges to better health in the Region (including the underlying root causes) through both rejuvenated work on public health and continued work on health systems;
2. improving governance in the WHO European Region and in the Regional Office;
3. further strengthening collaboration with Member States;
4. engaging in strategic partnerships for health and creating improved policy coherence;
5. strengthening the European contribution to global health;
6. reaching out through an information and communication strategy; and
7. promoting the Regional Office as an organization with a positive working environment and sustainable funding for its work.

Although each is important in itself, the priorities are related to each other and provide a framework or background for the rest of the Regional Office's work. Thus, the progress made on them is described more specifically in the next section and only summarized here. An examination of progress made towards the milestones set, however, shows that the vision for WHO in Europe is well on track to realization.

Progress towards the milestones in 2010–2011

The Regional Committee having set Europe's priorities in September 2010, the Regional Office and Member States started to work towards the milestones specified in their road map *(1)* and began to tackle the most urgent health issues in 2011, thus laying the foundation for the future. Between 2010 and 2011, the functions of the Regional Committee and SCRC were expanded and strengthened, and the Regional Office renewed its work as agreed with the Regional Committee. It reviewed its structures and its work in countries and developed a strategy on the latter. It made a plan for its human resources and pursued fundraising activities within the framework of the global strategy for resource mobilization.

Work to achieve the goal of developing a new European health policy, called Health 2020 *(5)*, along with supporting mechanisms, is well on track. In 2010–2011, the Regional Office started a development process seeking participation by and consultation with the widest possible range of stakeholders. This work included a new consultative body, the European Health Policy Forum of High-level Government Officials *(6)*, and the development of support mechanisms, including two studies (a European review of social determinants of health and the health divide *(7,8)* and a study on governance for health in the 21st century *(9)*), a limited number of targets and initiatives to strengthen public health in the Region *(10)*. The process will deliver both Health 2020 – in both long and short forms – and the support mechanisms to the 2012 Regional Committee for consideration.

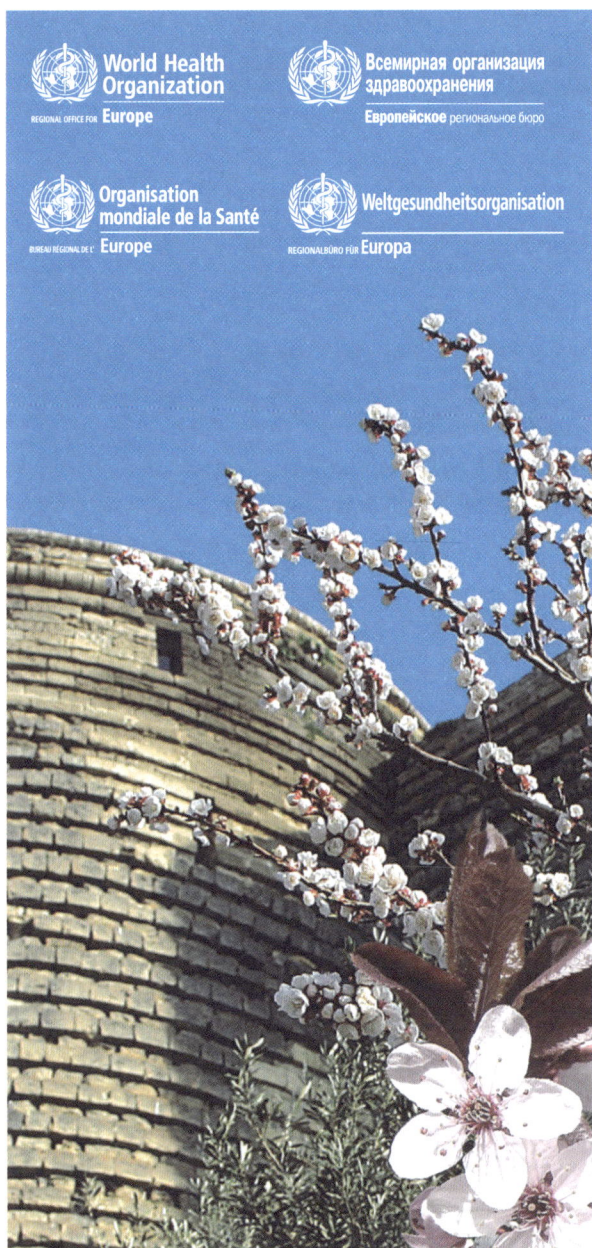
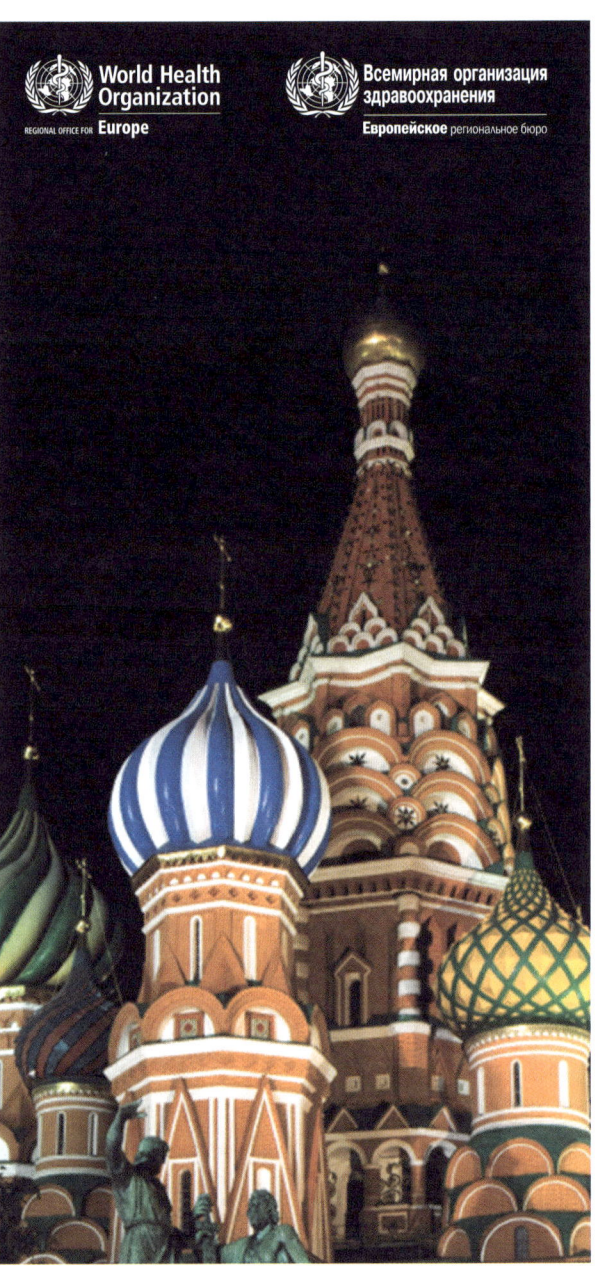

Even before completion, however, the Health 2020 process appeared to be building a new consensus between Member States on priorities in health. The 2011 Regional Committee agreed to make Region-wide responses to some pressing issues, adopting five action plans on: noncommunicable diseases, the harmful use of alcohol, HIV/AIDS, multidrug- and extensively drug-resistant tuberculosis, and antibiotic resistance (11–15). The first two were milestones on the road map, the alcohol action plan also demonstrating the Regional Office's renewed commitment to health promotion. Health 2020 provides a framework for not only the rest of the Regional Office's technical work but also policy development: the new action plans are similarly based on evidence and wide participation and consultation.

The Regional Office's work to strengthen its partnerships, particularly with the European Union (EU) but also with the Eurasian Economic Community, outstripped its efforts to craft a strategy on the topic. While the milestone of presenting such a strategy to the 2011 Regional Committee was postponed, the Regional Office and the European Commission made a historic declaration of strategic intent at the 2010 Regional Committee, quickly followed by choosing six areas for expanded cooperation and agreeing on the action to take in each *(16,17)*. The Regional Office also highlighted its work with partners at sessions of its governing bodies, and revitalized its networks, as shown by many examples in the following sections.

Finally, progress towards some milestones related to the functioning of the Regional Office was incomplete, due partially to the pressure of both other work and an additional opportunity on the 2011 Regional Committee. Although the Regional Office reviewed its work in countries and its geographically dispersed and country offices and prepared new strategies on them *(18,19)*, the pressure of other discussions – including lively and productive parallel sessions on WHO reform *(20)* – led the 2011 Regional Committee to defer consideration of them, as well as the new information and communication strategy for health. The Regional Office continued to refine these strategies after further consultation with Member States.

To sum up, a comparison of the progress described in this report with the aims of the seven strategic directions listed above shows that, as agreed by the Regional Office and Member States, WHO in Europe set its priorities in 2010 and took on some of the most pressing issues in 2011, thereby laying a foundation for the realization of its five-year vision.

About this report

This report presents WHO's work in Europe in 2010–2011 from two different directions. The next section examines overarching priorities of the Regional Office's work, while subsequent sections address particular technical areas. As the whole Office pursues the Regional Director's vision, these horizontal and vertical views overlap to some extent, although the report tries to keep this to a minimum.

While addressing the wide range of the Regional Office's work, this report does not present a detailed account of the implementation of technical programmes in the Region. That information is available from the Regional Office web site[1] and from the Secretariat upon request. This report concentrates on the major actions and changes implemented in the Regional Office in 2010–2011 and therefore presents highlights of its work. In addition, as the Regional Office works at three levels – global and interregional (including with WHO headquarters and other regional offices), and with countries at the regional or subregional level (including activities with networks) and individually (including with country offices) – most of the work described in this report involves activities on at least two of these levels.

---

[1] The web site (http://www.euro.who.int/en/home) provides information on the whole range of the Regional Office's work.

OVERARCHING PRIORITIES

In 2010–2011, the Regional Office pursued a number of overarching priorities, which were important both in themselves and as a framework or background for all its activities. This work can be discussed under the headings of the strategic priorities:

1. developing the new European health policy: Health 2020;
2. reinforcing governance of the WHO Regional Office for Europe;
3. reviewing Regional Office functions, offices and networks;
4. strengthening collaboration with Member States;
5. strengthening partnerships;
6. improving information and communication work;
7. creating a positive and empowering working environment and sustainable funding for the Regional Office.

New European health policy: Health 2020

In 2010, the Regional Office began a two-year participatory process to develop a new European health policy that would cover the period to 2020, provide an overarching framework for health development in Europe and guide all of the Regional Office's work *(21)*, including the new strategies and action plans described below. Health 2020 will call for a health-in-all-policies, whole-of-government and whole-of-society approach and use governance and health inequalities/social determinants as "lenses" through which to view all technical areas of health *(22)*.

The goal is to significantly improve the health and well-being of populations, to reduce health inequities and to ensure sustainable, people-centred health systems in order to achieve "a WHO European Region in which all people are enabled and supported in achieving their full health potential and well-being and in which countries, individually and jointly, work towards reducing inequities in health within the Region and beyond" *(5)*. Health 2020's strategic objectives are:

- stronger equity: working to improve health for all and reducing the health divide; and
- better governance: improving leadership and participatory governance for health.

And it has four common policy priorities:

- investing in health through a life-course approach and empowering people;
- tackling Europe's major health challenges: noncommunicable and communicable diseases;
- strengthening people-centred health systems and public health capacities, and emergency preparedness; and
- creating supportive environments and resilient communities.

Health 2020 will be a value-based action-oriented policy framework, adaptable to different realities in the countries in the European Region. It will address health ministries, but also aim to engage ministers and policy-makers across government and stakeholders throughout society, whose contribution to health and well-being is essential.

In developing the policy, the Regional Office both gathered evidence on which to base it and worked to consult and engage Member States and other partners. Thus, it conducted two major studies (a European review of social determinants of health and the health divide and a study on governance for health in the 21st century) and three investigations (on resolutions of the Regional Committee, the World Health Assembly and ministerial conferences, as well as conference declarations; the economics of disease prevention; and the experience gained with intersectoral work, notably in the European environment and health process since 1989 and in areas such as transport and obesity). Seeking discussion by and feedback from Member States, the Regional Office organized events to support the policy's development, including the first two meetings of the European Health Policy Forum of High-level Government Officials (see below) and a WHO conference on Health 2020 in November 2011, as well as putting it on the agendas of both the Regional Committee and SCRC (3,4,23–25). This work also included starting the development of a limited number of Health 2020 targets (26), and working to strengthen public health in the Region (see below).

First fruit of the process

By the start of 2012, the process was clearly bearing fruit, and Health 2020 was well on track for presentation to the 2012 Regional Committee in two forms:

- a short policy document aimed at policy-makers and governments as a whole, containing the key evidence, arguments and areas for policy action to address the public health challenges and the opportunities for promoting health and well-being in the European Region; and
- a longer policy framework and strategy aimed at the health and public health community at large, providing the contextual analysis and the main effective strategies and interventions, and describing the capacities necessary to implement the policy.

The final reports from the two major studies conducted to inform the new health policy for the Region will also be submitted to the Regional Committee in 2012, but both progressed well in 2010–2011. The first, the European review of social determinants of health and the health

Health 2020 documents

The short Health 2020 policy framework contains the **key evidence, arguments and areas for policy action** to address the public health challenges, and opportunities for promoting health and well-being in the European Region today.

The longer Health 2020 policy framework and strategy document provides the **contextual analysis and the main strategies and interventions** that work, and describes the necessary **capacities to implement** the policy.

divide, issued two interim reports *(7,8)*. The 2011 Regional Committee also received an interim report from the second: a comprehensive study of governance for health in the 21st century that made recommendations on how governments can strengthen governance for health through collaboration and described five smart governance approaches: synergistic, mixed, adaptable, respectful and transparent *(9)*.

In addition, the Regional Office's work on all the topics discussed in subsequent sections – such as fighting communicable and noncommunicable diseases, promoting health, strengthening health and public health systems, and creating supportive environments – are vital not only in themselves but also to Health 2020's four policy priorities.

Essential support: corporate functions

Governance and WHO reform

Efforts to improve the governance of the Regional Office were guided by the SCRC, included the adoption of a work package and resolution by the 2010 Regional Committee and continued through 2011 *(3,4,24,25)*. These included strengthening the Region's governing bodies: referring European policies, strategies and action plans for decision by the Regional Committee, making its programme more participatory for representatives and adding such events as ministerial panels and parallel working-group discussions. To cover a longer agenda, the sixty-first session of the Regional Committee was extended to four full days. To improve oversight and transparency, membership of the SCRC was increased from 9 to 12 countries in 2010, and all Member States were invited to attend the Eighteenth SCRC's fourth session; this session and a meeting of European delegations preceded the Sixty-fourth World Health Assembly in May 2011. In addition to reporting back on ministerial conferences to Regional Committee sessions, the Regional Office supported conferences in the Region: a European initiative on children with intellectual disabilities in November 2010, and a global conference on noncommunicable diseases in April 2011 (see below). The Regional Director ensured full accountability of the Regional Office to its governing bodies by reporting regularly to the SCRC on the implementation of the work programme.

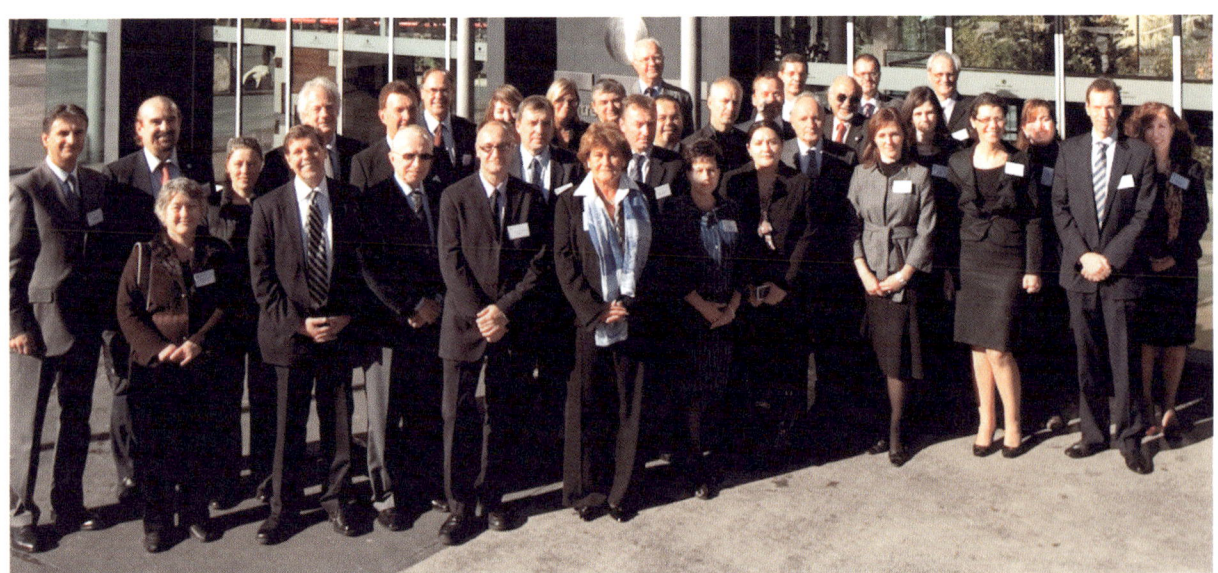

Overarching priorities

In addition, the Regional Office established the European Health Policy Forum of High-level Government Officials, to hold strategic discussions to facilitate consultation on Health 2020. The Forum, comprising delegations led by deputy health ministers and chief medical officers or similar high-level authorities, met twice in 2011, in Andorra in March and Israel in November (27). The participants discussed and advised on not only the development of Health 2020 but also such policy initiatives as the implementation of the Tallinn Charter (28), the strengthening of public health services and capacities, the European action plan on noncommunicable diseases, and the development of comprehensive national health policies and strategies.

The Regional Office also worked to enhance accountability for the decisions made by the Organization's governing bodies, both in WHO and in Member States, in order to focus attention on the common public health priorities of the Region, give donor Member States an improved framework for planning, ensure more predictable resources and link agreed outcomes with resources and performance. A pilot experiment was launched to attain these goals within the context of the WHO reform process (see below), endowing the budget with functional tools for transparency and accountability. The Regional Office would become more specifically accountable for the budget approved by the Regional Committee by taking responsibility for delivering key outputs, while Member States would be responsible for using them to improve population health. The Regional Office began operational planning for the 2012–2013 biennium in February 2011, presented a draft proposal to the SCRC in May and reported on progress in November (25).

Finally, the Regional Office participated fully in the WHO reform programme, launched at the start of 2011 by the Director-General, to make the Organization more flexible and effective. This included a plan to strengthen WHO's central role in global health governance, to strengthen its role as a directing and coordinating body of international health. The Region continued to participate in the reform process, both through the work of the Secretariat and in dedicated discussions during the 2011 session of the Regional Committee in which representatives gave their views on

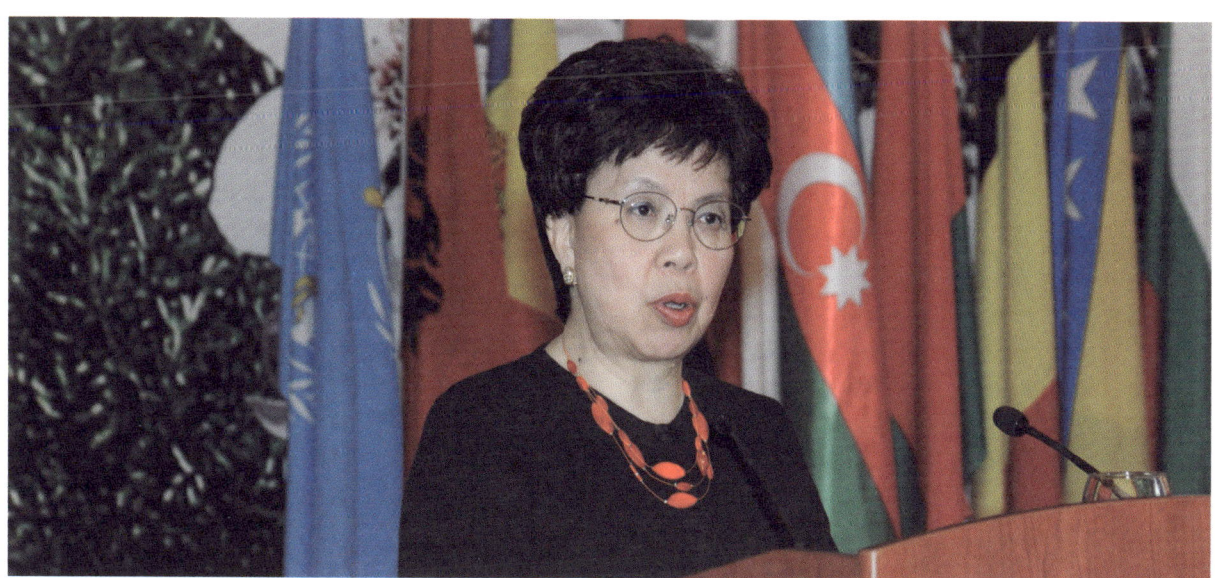

governance, core business and managerial reforms *(20)*. This information formed part of the Region's contribution to the WHO Executive Board special session on WHO reform in November *(29)*.

The Regional Director is fully committed to the global spirit of "one WHO" and supports the WHO Director-General in all her endeavours that serve this purpose, including the Global Policy Group, which comprises the WHO Director-General, the Deputy Director-General and regional directors. The European Region always follows up the decisions of WHO's global governing bodies.

Functions, offices and networks

In 2010–2011, the Regional Office worked to concentrate core corporate functions in the office in Copenhagen, fully integrate the geographically dispersed offices (GDOs) and country offices, and revitalize its networks. It conducted an in-depth analysis of its core functions and completed the reorganization aligning its structures and human resources with its new priorities. Staff were recruited (or seconded) to fill mission-critical senior technical positions to tackle the identified priorities.

To support decision-making about better integration of the GDOs and country offices in the Regional Office, the Regional Director set up two groups of external experts to conduct independent reviews. In November 2010, both reported their findings. The Regional Office incorporated these in its new strategies on GDOs *(19)* and work with countries (see below). The review group on GDOs found that the four in operation – addressing health systems (Barcelona, Spain), environment and health (Bonn, Germany and Rome, Italy) and investment for health (Venice, Italy) – not only did excellent work but also served as a fund-raising mechanism for the Regional Office. The group recommended strengthening direction by and coordination within the Regional Office, improving GDOs' funding and balancing their work between intercountry activities and direct assistance to countries, and establishing new GDOs. The group's findings were incorporated in the renewed strategy on GDOs that will be presented to the Regional Committee in 2012 *(19)*.

In September 2011, the finalization of the host agreement on the new GDO on noncommunicable diseases was celebrated in Athens, Greece; it was agreed that the recruitment of the staff for the GDO would start when the schedule and release of payments were confirmed. Owing to a change in the Italian Government's priorities and the consequent ceasing of its support for the Rome Office *(30)*, however, the Regional Office closed it and, with support from the German Government, consolidated European work on environment and health in the Bonn Office, while maintaining a strong policy and managerial base at the head office in Copenhagen, in line with the recommendations of the GDO review group and strategy *(19,31)*. The consolidation process was completed by January 2012.

The World Health Assembly's new policy on partnerships *(32)*, as well as the Regional Committee's decision to keep core functions at the head office in Copenhagen, along with the intention to further promote partnerships, necessitated a review of the governance of the European Observatory on Health Systems and Policies *(33)*. The Regional Office led the process and consulted with the Observatory's partner organizations to reach these objectives and to complete the work during 2011.

In 2010–2011, the South-eastern Europe Health Network (SEEHN) continued to set an example of the benefits of cooperation between WHO, other partners and countries in a part of the European Region. Since its creation in 2001, SEEHN, with strong support from the Regional Office and the Council of Europe, had been the undisputed vehicle for health development in its member countries: Albania, Bosnia and Herzegovina, Bulgaria, Croatia, Montenegro, the Republic of Moldova, Romania, Serbia and the former Yugoslav Republic of Macedonia. In November 2010, the nine members signed the first multicountry legal agreement on public health in south-eastern Europe, turning a WHO network for regional cooperation into an independent legal entity. SEEHN member countries opened several regional health development centres: inaugurating a centre on organ donation and transplantation in Croatia in February 2011, and those on mental health in Bosnia and Herzegovina and on antibiotic resistance in Bulgaria in June.

Along with the Council of Europe and donor countries, the Regional Office continued to support SEEHN, including its third health ministers' forum in Banja Luka, Bosnia and Herzegovina in October 2011 *(34)*. At the Forum, SEEHN welcomed a new member, Israel, and ministers signed the Banja Luka Pledge, expressing political commitment to extending regional cooperation to introduce and/or strengthen the values, priorities and action needed to achieve equity and accountability in health *(35)*.

Collaboration with Member States

The working group to review strategic relations with countries identified both strengths and weaknesses in the Regional Office's current arrangements for country work. To improve this work, the group recommended that the Regional Office:

- strengthen its technical capacity;
- develop a new country strategy;
- use one set of criteria to determine the type of presence and level of institutional support needed, ranging from a full country office, through a smaller country-cooperation office to a desk officer at the Regional Office;
- explore new mechanisms to ensuring the exchange of experience and information through improved intercountry work; and
- if it proved successful, roll out the pilot scheme to replace biennial collaborative agreements (BCAs) with country cooperation strategies across the Region.

The Regional Office developed a new strategy on work with countries for presentation to the 2011 Regional Committee *(18)*, drawing on the work

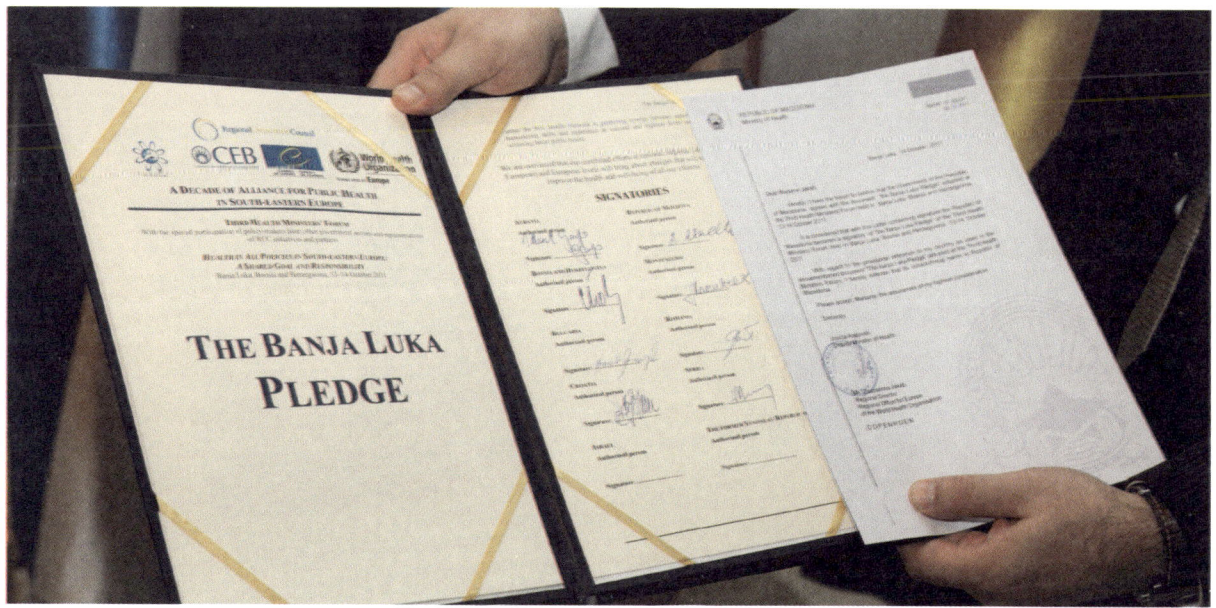

of the external review group. The strategy aims to ensure that, by adopting a holistic and coherent approach, WHO is relevant to every Member State in the diverse European Region, and it emphasizes coordinating and streamlining activities and making full use of existing resources in countries. As discussion by the Regional Committee was delayed until 2012 (see above), the Regional Office took the opportunity to continue refining the strategy, including aligning it with the outcomes of the discussion of WHO reform. It planned three subregional consultations for early 2012 and started developing an action plan and road map for implementing the strategy. The action plan would provide an evidence-based approach to restructuring the country offices.

Intensive collaboration with Member States continued; it emphasized supporting countries in their most important health developments (strengthening national policy and health systems) while providing continued support to high-priority technical areas. The Regional Office pursued this task through two different kinds of structures.

Country offices worked to carry out BCAs between the Regional Office and host countries. A dedicated programme in the head office in Copenhagen not only organized collaboration with other Member States but also liaised between technical programmes and country offices in the planning and signing of BCAs for 2012–2013 and arranged for health ministers to visit the Regional Office to learn more about its work and strengthen its cooperation with their countries.

The Regional Office started a new initiative to explore with European Member States their interest in developing country cooperation strategies with WHO, as part of the WHO reform process.

Partnerships

While partnerships have always been at the forefront of its work, in 2010–2011 the Regional Office sought to improve relations and foster cooperation with a wide range of partners: the EU and its institutions, the United Nations system, subregional networks, global health partnerships, the private sector and philanthropic foundations, and civil-society

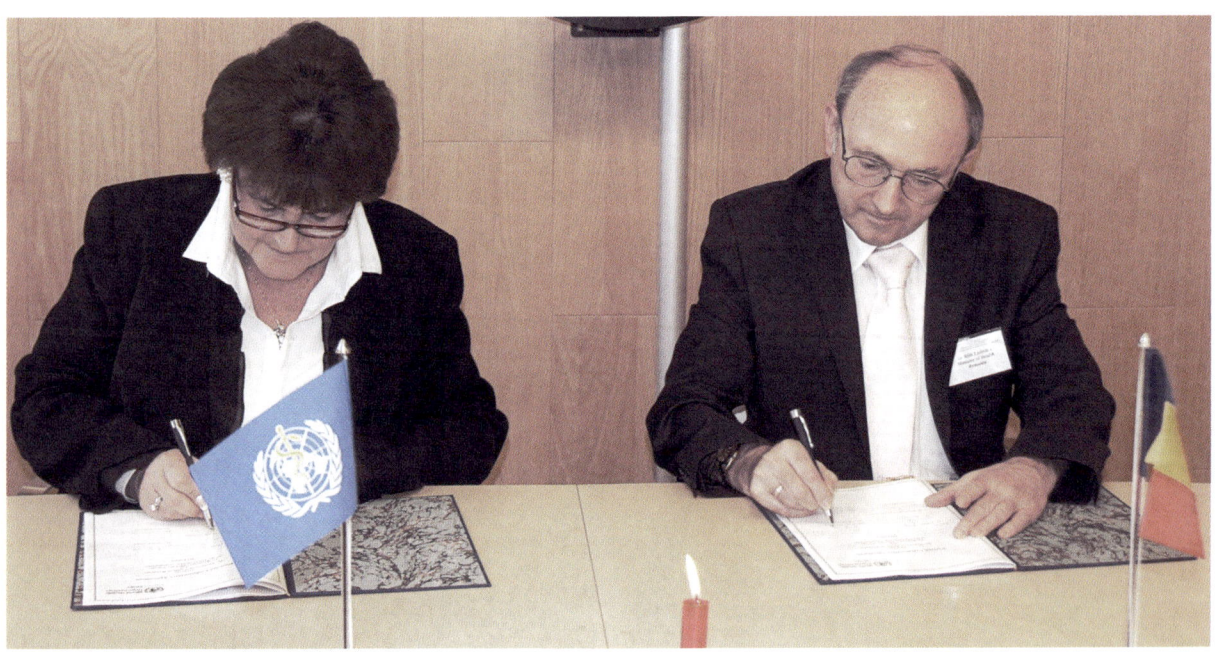

organizations. Examples of this cooperation abound throughout this report. Although the Regional Office intended to develop a strategy on partnerships for submission to the Regional Committee, the need to align it with WHO reforms led the SCRC to agree that development needed to await the completion of the reform process *(25)*.

At the request of the Director-General and the Global Policy Group, the Regional Director agreed to coordinate collaboration between the EU and WHO globally and to establish and chair a WHO steering group on the EU, respectively. The Regional Office and the European Commission (EC) put into effect the joint declaration launched by the WHO Regional Director for Europe and the European Commissioner for Health and Consumers at the 2010 session of the Regional Committee *(16)*. At the annual meeting of senior officials from WHO and EC, as well as a high-level meeting in Brussels, Belgium in March 2011, the partners agreed on global strategic cooperation in six areas: health security, health innovation, health systems, health information, health inequalities and in-country collaboration, and they finalized road maps for implementing the commitments in the joint declaration. *(17)*. Later sections give many examples of joint work in these areas.

In addition, the Regional Office and the European Centre for Disease Prevention and Control (ECDC) signed an administrative agreement in March 2011 and established a joint coordination group to follow up its implementation (see below). Continuing collaboration includes joint publications, meetings and consultations with ECDC to strengthen coordinated surveillance of tuberculosis, HIV and influenza, and support the implementation of the International Health Regulations (IHR). The partners made plans to expand this cooperation into shared regional surveillance of measles and rubella, and to use the EC surveillance system for monitoring antimicrobial resistance (AMR) as a model for expanding AMR surveillance capacity into non-EU Member States. Several joint risk assessment missions were carried out during the year in response to disease outbreaks and other public health incidents.

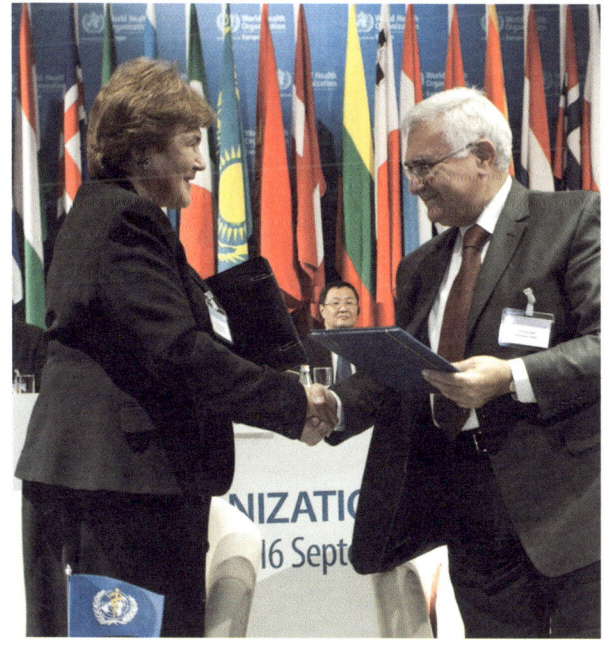

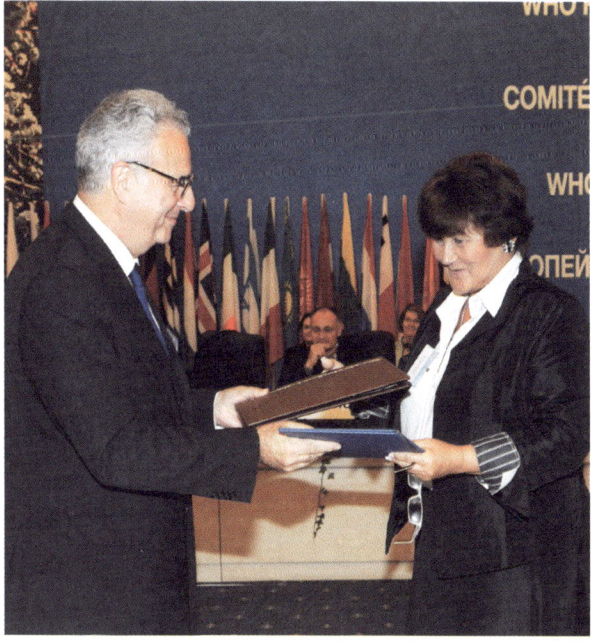

In 2010–2011, the Regional Office supported the health priorities of and expanded cooperation with the countries holding or preparing to hold the Presidency of the Council of the European Union (Belgium, Hungary, Poland and Denmark), and staff took part in hearings at the European Parliament. It also sought to strengthen its links with other members of the United Nations family and international agencies through, for example, active participation in meetings of the United Nations regional directors team and meetings with staff of the World Bank and the Organisation for Economic Co-operation and Development (OECD). At the 2011 session of the Regional Committee, the Regional Office and the Global Fund to Fight AIDS, Tuberculosis and Malaria initiated a joint operational plan for 2011–2012, in letters exchanged by the Regional Director and the Fund's Executive Director.

Partnership is essential to most Regional Office activities; for example, it consulted bodies such as the European Public Health Association (EUPHA), the Association of Schools of Public Health in the European Region (ASPHER), the European Forum of Medical Associations, the World Medical Association (WMA), the European Forum of National Nursing and Midwifery Associations and the European Health Forum Gastein, as well as a wide range of nongovernmental organizations (NGOs), on Health 2020 and other issues. The Regional Office also strengthened its work with the network of WHO collaborating centres: for example, several contributed technical expertise to the response to environmental and man-made emergencies (see below). In addition, it actively participated in major events held by partners, such as many meetings organized by holders of the EU Presidency, the World Health Summit in October 2010 and the European Health Forum Gastein. Further, the Regional Office continued its partnerships within WHO, including work with other regional offices on disease surveillance and control and on harmonization of country work (hosting the tenth global meeting of country

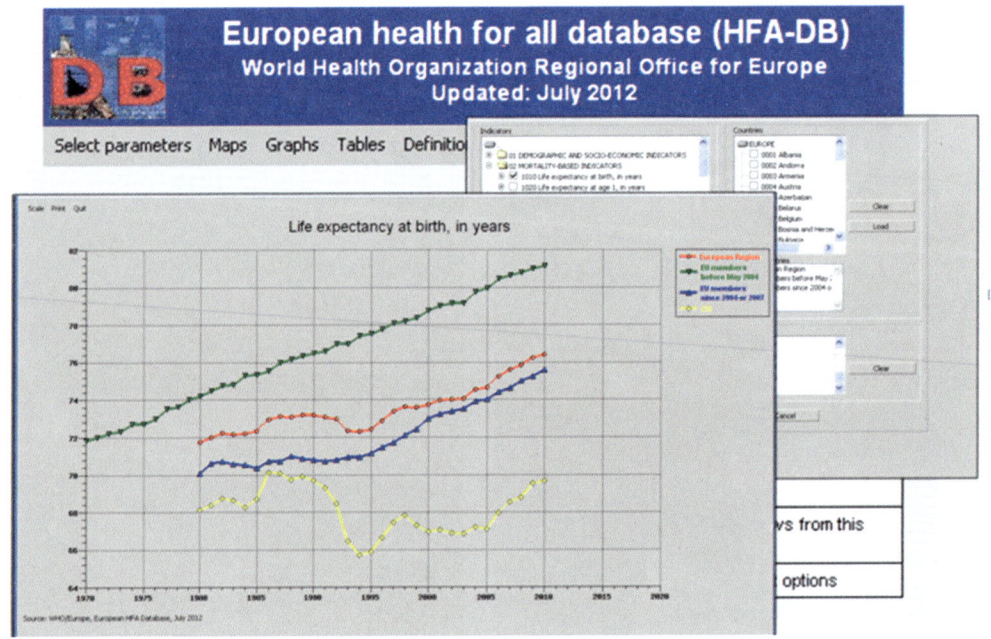

support units), as well as work in the Global Policy Group on planning and implementing WHO reform and other global matters.

Finally, distinguished public personalities, including Her Royal Highness Crown Princess Mary of Denmark, Patron of the Regional Office, helped the Regional Office to promote public health in the European Region. Mrs Sandra Roelofs, the First Lady of Georgia, WHO Goodwill Ambassador for the Health-related Millennium Development Goals in the European Region, visited the Regional Office in March 2011, and Her Royal Highness Princess Mathilde of Belgium helped launch European Immunization Week in April 2011 (see below).

Information and communication

Information and communication are vital elements in nearly all activities. The Regional Office not only provides information for both technical audiences and policy-makers (see below) but also uses both traditional and new media to publicize its work and to consult with a range of stakeholders.

The Regional Office set up an internal statistical policy group; in 2011 it inventoried and reviewed all the Office's databases and their associated indicators, including the Health for All database, one of the Regional Office's most widely used information products (36). They comprise the most comprehensive and authoritative source of health information available to policy-makers, stakeholders and the general public throughout the Region. The group's next task was to use the resulting information to streamline all databases, and thus take the first step towards building a unified Regional Office health information platform.

The Regional Office aligned its communications activities to support the vision outlined in this report. It implemented many projects to support technical programmes and Member States, including issuing 55 press releases between September 2010 and January 2012 (37). To boost efficiency and cohesion,

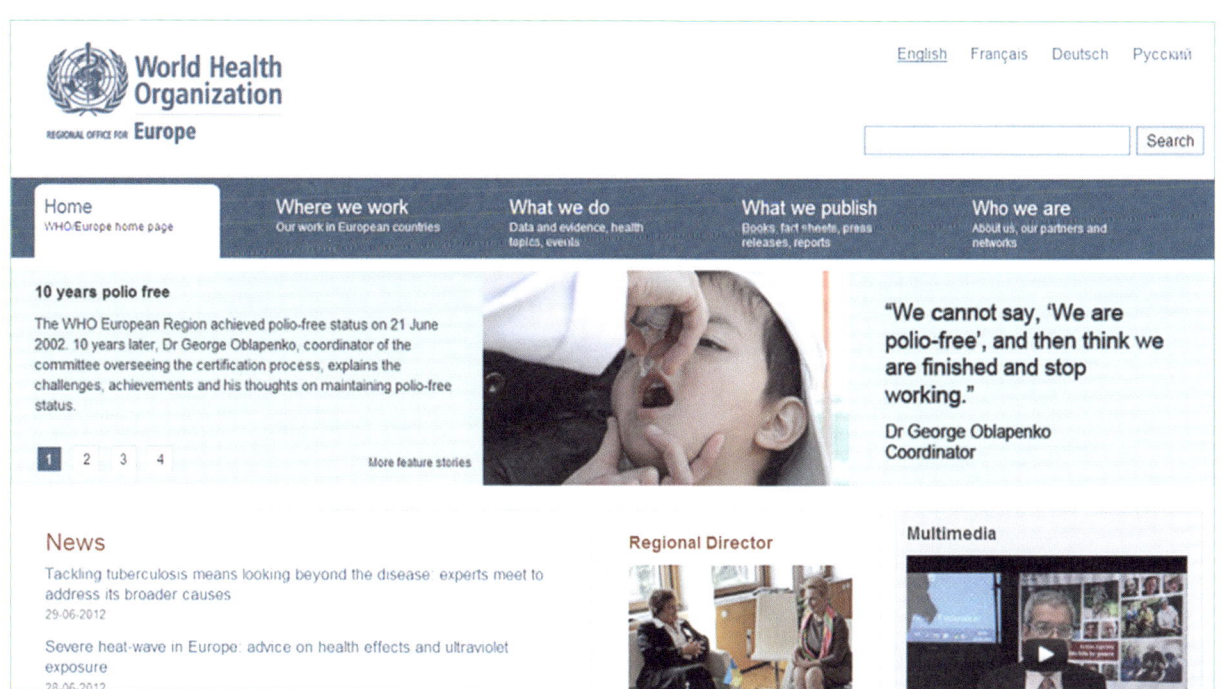

the Regional Office implemented a comprehensive internal communications strategy, optimizing the use of its intranet as a key platform and increasing information sharing and interaction between all regional offices. It used new and innovative methods, including social media, to encourage dialogue with key audiences and add transparency to its policy-development and norm-setting work.

The Regional Office used social media for online consultations on regional and global health priorities, such as Health 2020, WHO reform, the country strategy, and the action plans on HIV/AIDS and drug-resistant tuberculosis (see below). It developed an active presence on Facebook, Twitter and other platforms. The Regional Committee sessions in 2010 and 2011 as well as other high-level meetings were streamed live on the web and documented in detail through photos, videos and reports *(3,4,24,25)*, supporting Member States and making their decision-making more transparent and accessible. For European Immunization Week and World No Tobacco Day 2011, for example, the Regional Office worked through a range of media, including specially designed campaign sites *(38)*, and made podcasts and videos available to the public through various channels.

The web site remained the Regional Office's primary tool for communication and dissemination of policy-making and technical information in the four official languages, although it was relaunched with a new structure and updated content in May 2010, to reflect the new vision and priorities. For example, the frequently asked questions and updates on an outbreak of enterohaemorrhagic *Escherichia coli* infection in Germany (see below) received over 100 000 page views in one week in June 2011. Electronic dissemination of publications dwarfed hard-copy dissemination: the 10 most popular were downloaded almost 35 000 times annually.

Finally, the Regional Office developed strategies on communication and information for submission to the Regional Committee in 2012. The last section of this report gives details on more information activities.

Empowering working environment and sustainable funding

The Regional Office established an internal committee for a productive and healthy work environment. Working with the Staff Association, the Ombudspersons and other initiatives in the Office, the committee sought to identify common problems, practicable improvements and concrete steps to take; to formulate a road map with clear steps and time frame; and to facilitate implementation of approved recommendations.

In line with the global strategy for resource mobilization, the Regional Office's work to ensure greater accountability through the programme budget for 2012–2013 aimed to ensure sustainable funding for the most important priorities *(39)*. The European Region's proposed programme budget amounted to US$ 213 million; 27 key priority outcomes were identified for specific follow-up. For advocacy and fund-raising purposes, the Regional Office issued 11 booklets *(40)* describing its technical work with Member States, according to WHO's strategic objectives for 2008–2013. The Annex gives information on the budget for and spending in 2010–2011.

COMMUNICABLE DISEASES

The Regional Office's work shows evidence both of the successes achieved and of the challenges faced in communicable disease prevention and control and health security in the WHO European Region.

HIV/AIDS

While the rest of the world observed annual decreases in the number of new HIV cases in 2010, new infections increased by 18% in the European Region: from 6.6 per 100 000 population in 2004 to 7.8 in 2010 in the 50 countries that consistently reported HIV surveillance data over the period *(41)*. In eastern Europe and central Asia between 2001 and 2010, the number of people estimated to be living with HIV tripled and the number of those dying from AIDS-related causes increased more than tenfold from 7 800 to 90 000. The burden of HIV in the Region is unevenly distributed both between and within countries, falling most heavily on eastern countries and on groups of people who are socially marginalized and whose behaviour is socially stigmatized or illegal, such as sex workers and people who inject drugs. The incarceration of people in these groups also accelerates the spread of HIV in the Region.

To address this situation, the Regional Office prepared a European Action Plan for HIV/AIDS that the Regional Committee adopted in 2011 *(13)*. The Plan was developed through a consultative process and with the broad involvement of Member States, the SCRC, civil society, donor and development agencies, NGOs,

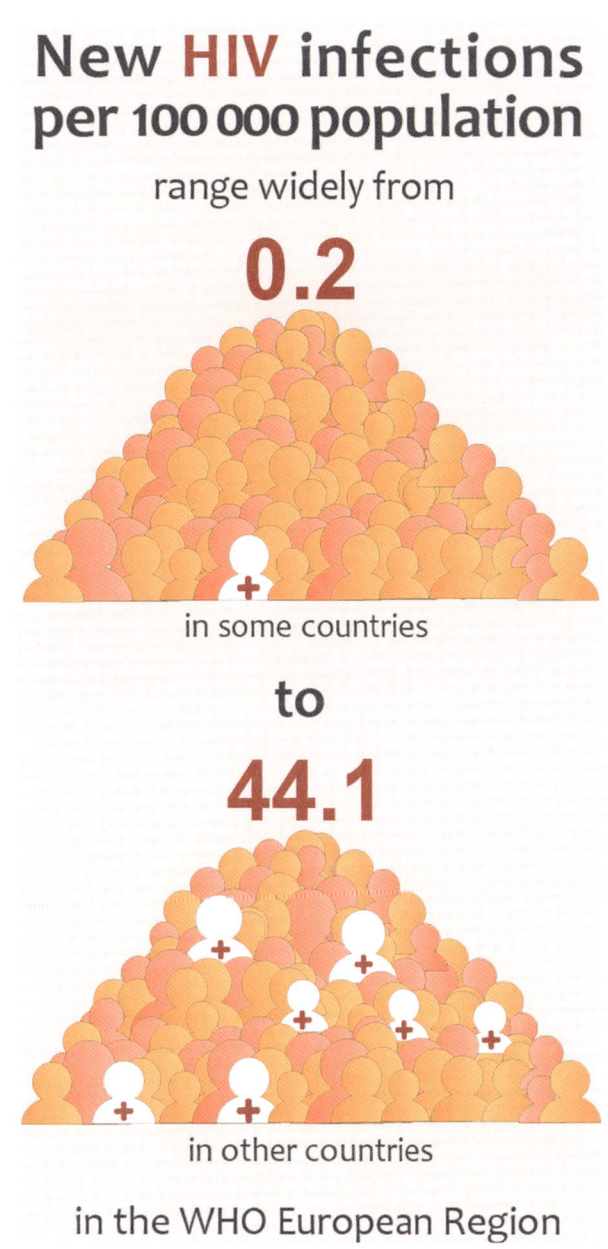

multilateral agencies, the Joint United Nations Programme on HIV/AIDS (UNAIDS) and co-sponsors, and EC scientific and technical institutions. It calls for the spread of HIV in the Region to be halted and reversed, and for universal access to HIV prevention, diagnosis, treatment and care to be achieved, by 2015.

The Plan also takes account of and builds on regional priorities within the context of such policy guidance as WHO's global health sector strategy on HIV and the UNAIDS strategy 2011–2015: "Getting to Zero" *(42,43)*, as well as the broader framework of the United Nations Millennium Development Goals (MDGs), particularly MDG 6 on combating HIV/AIDS. It is coherent with the EC communication on HIV/AIDS 2009–2013 and fully aligned with the Political Declaration endorsed at the United Nations high-level meeting on HIV/AIDS, held in New York in June 2011 *(44,45)*. The Plan was officially launched in London, United Kingdom and Moscow, Russian Federation in November 2011. With the support of the Global Fund to Fight AIDS, Tuberculosis and Malaria to eligible countries, the Regional Office supported Member States to implement the Plan and began collecting baseline data to monitor progress.

94% of TB deaths occurred in 34% of the countries in the European Region

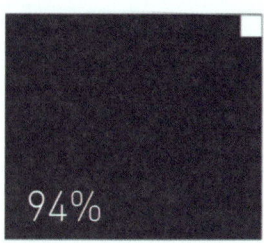
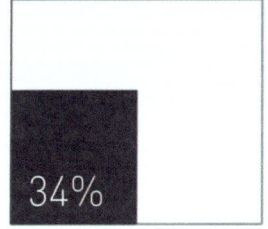

Tuberculosis

Drug-resistant tuberculosis (TB) and the spread of TB/HIV co-infections are significant public health concerns in Europe. In the WHO European Region alone, TB makes 42 people ill and kills 7 every hour. While the Region accounted for only 5.6% of newly detected and relapsed TB cases in the world, it reported over 300 000 new episodes of TB in 2010 with almost 39 000 deaths. The 18 high-priority countries for TB (countries in eastern Europe and central Asia, Bulgaria, Romania and Turkey) had notification rates for newly detected and relapsed TB cases almost eight times those in the rest of the Region; these countries also accounted for 94% of TB deaths in the entire Region and most of the increases in HIV co-infections and in multidrug- and extensively drug-resistant TB (M/XDR-TB) cases *(46)*.

In response to this alarming problem, the Regional Director established a special project to prevent and control M/XDR-TB in the Region. Under its framework, particular attention is paid to previously neglected childhood TB, and the Regional Office hosts a task force to review and adapt international guidelines and assist Member States in preventing and controlling TB and MDR-TB in children.

To scale up a comprehensive response and to prevent and control M/XDR-TB in the WHO European Region, the Regional Office prepared and the 2011 Regional Committee adopted the Consolidated Action Plan to Prevent and Combat Multidrug- and Extensively Drug-resistant Tuberculosis in the WHO European Region 2011–2015 *(14)*. It was developed through a broad consultation with Member States and other partners, experts, civil society and communities. It has six cross-cutting strategic directions, designed to foster the values of Health 2020, and seven areas of intervention. The latter are also aligned with the Global Plan to Stop TB 2011–2015 *(47)* and take account of World Health Assembly resolution WHA62.15 *(48)*, which urges Member States to prevent and control M/XDR-TB, strengthen partnership (for example, with the Global Fund), involve civil-society organizations and provide universal access to diagnosis and treatment. In addition, the Regional Office published a detailed road map, along with a monitoring and evaluation framework, for implementation of the Plan *(49)*. The budget was prepared with the assistance of a Dutch partnership and in collaboration with the Royal Tropical Institute in Amsterdam, the Netherlands. It also began to assist countries to adopt and harmonize their national health strategies or national responses to M/XDR-TB with the Action Plan.

In response to the need to scale up programmatic management of drug-resistant TB and provide advice to donors, the Regional Office for Europe was the first in WHO to have established and to host a regional Green Light Committee *(50)*. It explores mechanisms for advocating efforts to prevent and combat M/XDR-TB, and assists Member States in developing and implementing participatory and inclusive plans to address MDR-TB. In addition, the Regional Office reviewed the TB programmes in countries (Armenia, Belarus, Denmark (Greenland), Estonia, Finland, Kyrgyzstan, Latvia, Norway, Turkmenistan and Uzbekistan) and recommended improvements, and surveyed resistance to anti-TB drugs in Azerbaijan, Belarus, the Russian Federation, Turkmenistan, Ukraine and Uzbekistan, and with ECDC for the EU.

Malaria

The WHO European Region made remarkable progress against malaria in 2010–2011. The number of reported locally acquired cases dropped dramatically: from 90 712 in 1995 to only 102 in 2011 in Azerbaijan, Georgia, Tajikistan and Turkey and including a small-scale outbreak in Greece. Turkmenistan and Armenia were certified as malaria free in 2010 and 2011, respectively; Kazakhstan began the certification process and Georgia was preparing for it *(51)*. This very encouraging progress suggests that the Region is on course to meet the Tashkent Declaration's goal of eliminating malaria from the WHO European Region by 2015 *(52)*.

Nevertheless, an increase in mosquito-borne diseases, including malaria, West Nile fever, dengue and Chikungunya, was noted in summer 2011.

Vaccine-preventable diseases and immunization

Sustaining polio-free status

In 2010–2011, the European Region responded to its first outbreak of poliomyelitis (polio), following importation of poliovirus, since certification as polio free in 2002. The outbreak caused severe harm to health: 475 cases were reported (457 cases in Tajikistan, 14 in the Russian Federation, 3 in Turkmenistan and 1 in Kazakhstan), resulting in 30 deaths *(53)*. It also threatened the European Region's polio-free status.

In 2010–2011, the Regional Office assisted affected countries in their responses and worked to keep Europe polio free. With its support, Kazakhstan, Kyrgyzstan, the Russian Federation, Tajikistan, Turkmenistan and Uzbekistan conducted several rounds of supplemental immunization activities (SIAs) between May and December 2010 vaccinating more than 22 million children. Azerbaijan conducted subnational SIAs in areas bordering the Russian Federation in spring 2011 and Georgia conducted mop-up activities in May–June 2011, targeting children who had not completed polio vaccination schedules.

Meeting in the Russian Federation in January 2011, the European Regional Certification Commission for Poliomyelitis Eradication (RCC) commended the affected countries on their response to the outbreak, and noted the need to address long-term structural and system issues. The countries presented their epidemiological situations and response measures for review. Meeting in Copenhagen in August 2011, the RCC recognized that Member States had adopted its recommendations, concluded that countries had provided sufficient evidence on immunization coverage and the sensitivity of their polio surveillance systems, and announced that Europe would retain its polio-free status. The RCC also acknowledged the contributions and technical support of the WHO Regional Office for Europe, the partners in the Global Polio Eradication Initiative, the Russian Federation, India and the United States Agency for International Development (USAID) *(54)*.

In the midst of the polio outbreak, an online laboratory tool was introduced for the regional polio laboratory network. This tool proved very useful in streamlining reporting and making it more accessible, so the Regional Office created an improved version of the tool – the Online Laboratory Data Management System – and launched it in March 2011 *(55)*.

In February 2011, WHO, the United Nations Children's Fund (UNICEF), Operation Mercy (OM) and Handicap International (HI) launched a training initiative to provide long-term rehabilitation to address the needs of more than 400 people in Tajikistan, paralysed due to wild poliovirus (not confined to cases contracted during the most recent outbreak).

Measles and rubella elimination

In 2010, the Regional Committee endorsed a new target date (2015) for the elimination of measles and rubella *(3)*. Both continued to spread across the European Region, however, causing large outbreaks in a number of western European countries. There was particular concern about outbreaks of rubella in Romania and measles in Ukraine, with more than 34 000 confirmed measles cases and nearly 4 000 suspected rubella cases in 2011, respectively. The Regional Office continued to work closely with countries, providing recommendations as needed (such as adding an additional dose of measles vaccine at 6 months of age during the outbreaks) and issued monthly reports on the situation and response *(53)*. The Regional Office started the elimination-verification process and developed a framework to document progress *(56)*.

Current outbreaks clearly resulted from a failure to vaccinate, not the failure of measles vaccine. All available information, official and unofficial, confirmed that most of the reported cases were not immunized against measles. This was not a problem confined to specific countries or subregions, and all

Communicable diseases

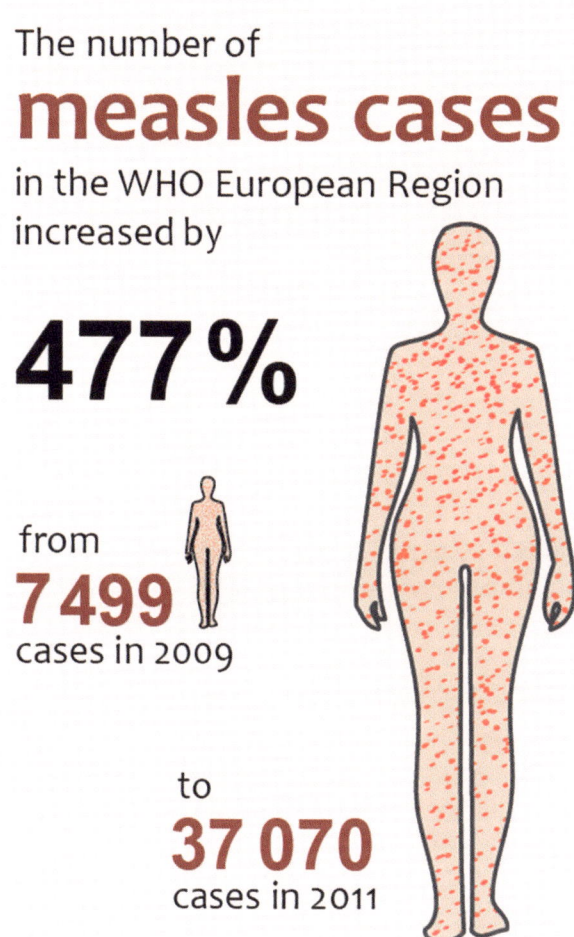

The number of **measles cases** in the WHO European Region increased by **477%** from **7 499** cases in 2009 to **37 070** cases in 2011

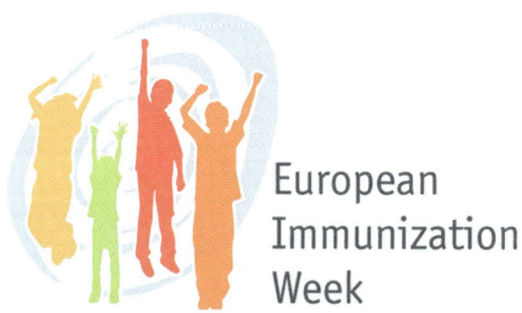

European Immunization Week
Prevent Protect Immunize

Member States were obviously at risk of outbreaks. Further, measles was exported from countries with outbreaks to other countries in the Region and to other regions of the world.

European Immunization Week

The annual European Immunization Week (EIW) is a success, growing from 6 participating countries in 2005 to 52 in 2011. Against the backdrop of the polio outbreak in 2010 and the ongoing challenge of measles in 2011, EIW provided Member States with an important opportunity to advocate immunization and, in some cases, to conduct outreach activities and SIAs.

The Regional Office held its sixth EIW from 23 to 30 April 2011 (38,57). The theme of "shared solutions to common threats" focused on the recent and ongoing outbreaks in the Region and how subregions could work together to respond to such events and prevent further outbreaks. Regional and national partners, including UNICEF and ECDC, supported implementation. Many influential people and organizations made statements supporting EIW, including Her Royal Highness Crown Princess Mary of Denmark; Her Royal Highness Princess Mathilde of Belgium, the Office's Special Representative for Immunization; Mr Bill Gates, co-chair of the Bill and Melinda Gates Foundation; the GAVI Alliance; and Professor David M. Salisbury, Chair of the RCC. A regional launch was held in Brussels, followed by a round-table discussion with high-level officials from Belgium, France, Germany and Switzerland, to review the continuing measles outbreaks and to share best practices in control measures.

EIW 2011 was the most successful to date, with participation from 52 of the Region's Member States (only 6 countries took part in the first EIW in 2005). More than 25 countries launched media outreach campaigns, including press conferences and releases, workshops and interviews given by public health officials. More than 25 countries also developed and implemented information campaigns, using traditional printed materials and innovative communication tools on the Internet and mobile telephones. Several countries implemented immunization campaigns, often using mobile immunization teams and engaging in field visits to determine immunization status *(57)*.

Strengthening routine immunization services and introducing new vaccines

In 2011 the Regional Office conducted research to develop strategies and interventions to help Member States reach the un- and under-vaccinated children in the Region. It worked to strengthen training in the Region by building sustainable institutional capacity in countries. The Regional Office held training courses on mid-level management and immunization in practice. It also worked closely with WHO headquarters to improve access to data and information on vaccine prices, procurement and product characteristics, to enable countries to make informed decisions on the financially sustainable use of current and new vaccines. To increase countries' ownership of immunization programmes, the Regional Office worked to develop comprehensive multiyear plans in 2011, and to set up and strengthen national immunization advisory groups, particularly in low- and lower-middle-income countries.

The Regional Office assisted low-income countries in decision-making and collecting the surveillance and economic data that allow them to make informed decisions on introducing new vaccines. It also provided technical support for evaluations before and after introduction. In 2011, the Regional Office worked with Armenia, Georgia, and the Republic of Moldova to prepare their immunization programmes for the introduction of rotavirus vaccines in the first half of 2012. This assisted the countries in securing funding from the GAVI Alliance. The Regional Office organized a meeting in October 2011 in Istanbul, Turkey at which over 40 countries reviewed their progress and shared experience, best practices and lessons learned about preventing cervical cancer, which is almost entirely caused by the vaccine-preventable human papillomavirus (HPV).

Influenza

The Regional Office worked for pandemic preparedness and on seasonal influenza surveillance jointly with ECDC, published regular bulletins on influenza in the Region and updated its guidance on sentinel surveillance *(58,59)*. The partners held their first joint annual regional meeting for influenza surveillance in Slovenia in June 2011, stressing the importance of continuing to work on influenza after the pandemic. Between September and November 2011, the Regional Office and ECDC organized four workshops that helped countries revise their pandemic preparedness plans by summarizing the key changes being made and enabling countries to learn from each other's experience; 45 countries participated *(60)*.

The Regional Office continued to support capacity building among national influenza centres (NICs) by providing on-site assessment, training and quality-assurance programmes. In 2010, it recognized the NIC in Malta; 40 countries had a WHO-recognized NIC. In addition, using surveillance data provided by countries, the Regional Office showed that, compared to seasonal influenza, the 2009 pandemic had caused a significantly higher number of outpatient consultations in children in most countries and followed the west-to-east spread previously observed during some influenza seasons *(61)*.

In December 2010, the Regional Office reported on its multicountry evaluation of the response to pandemic (H1N1) 2009 influenza *(62)*. The evaluation involved a broad range of stakeholders at the national, regional and local levels in seven

Communicable diseases

countries selected randomly across the Region. Interviews were conducted with representatives from health and civil-response ministries, national public health authorities, regional authorities, general practitioners and hospital physicians, and the results were analysed and discussed during a workshop involving all stakeholders, in Copenhagen in October 2010. The evaluation also took account of the report and recommendations of the independent Review Committee on the Functioning of the International Health Regulations, which identified the lessons learnt during the global response to the pandemic in order to strengthen the functioning of the IHR, the continuing global response (including the role of WHO) and preparedness for future pandemics *(63)*. This work contributed to the endorsement of the Pandemic Influenza Preparedness Framework for the sharing of influenza viruses and access to vaccines and other benefits, adopted by the 2011 World Health Assembly *(64)*.

Also in 2010, the Regional Office worked with the Member States who received donated pandemic influenza vaccine to administer the vaccine through campaigns targeting particular populations. In collaboration with an ECDC project, it made the first survey of policies on and uptake of seasonal influenza vaccine in 2011, to measure progress towards the 2005 WHO target of 75% vaccine coverage of elderly people. In addition, the Regional Office provided regular updates on vaccine safety issues and addressed Member States' specific questions on safety and vaccine procurement.

After the 2009–2010 pandemic, WHO developed guidance for health care providers on the clinical management of influenza *(65)*.

Antimicrobial resistance

At present, 25 000 people die in the EU every year because of a serious resistant bacterial infection, mostly acquired in health care settings. In addition to causing deaths and increased suffering, antimicrobial resistance (AMR) has huge economic implications.

This emerging health threat was the focus of World Health Day 2011, with the slogan "Antibiotic resistance: No action today, no cure tomorrow" *(66)*. To mark World Health Day and raise awareness, the Regional Office organized and supported a number of key activities and press events across the European

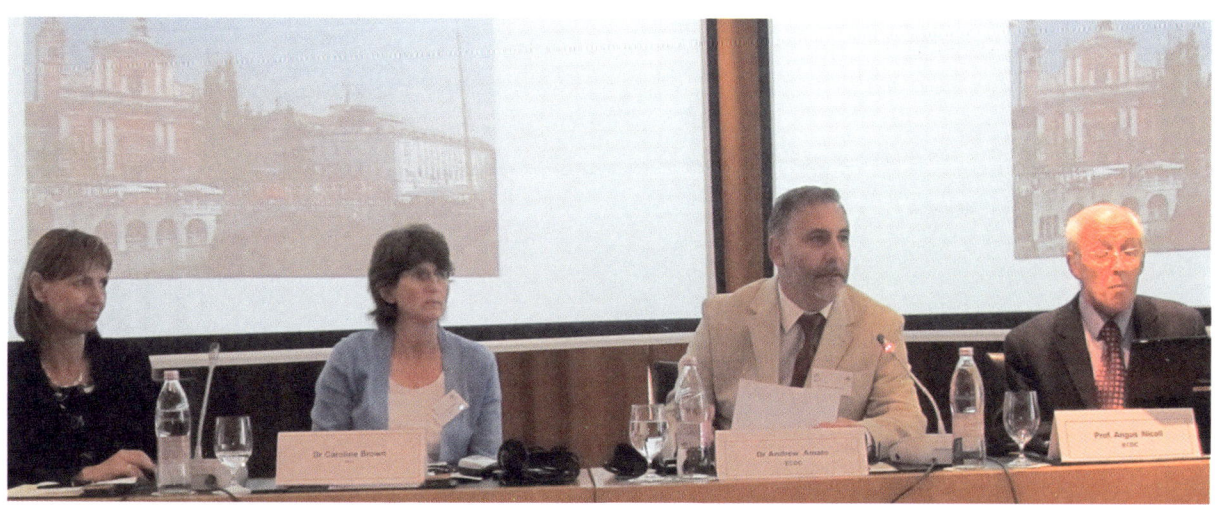

Region, in Moscow, Strasbourg, Copenhagen, Rome and London, for example. It also published a successful book on antibiotic resistance from a food safety perspective *(67)*.

AMR is driven by complex factors and should be addressed through joint action by a wide range of stakeholders and partners, implementing national, regional and global policies based on public health principles. Countries need to exercise all-inclusive national cooperation to develop, guide and monitor national action plans involving all stakeholders and sectors.

In this context and in addition to the AMR strategies launched by the EU and WHO in 2000 and 2001, respectively, the Regional Office developed a regional strategic action plan on antibacterial resistance *(15)*, with seven strategic objectives that promote an integrated and comprehensive approach; it focuses mainly on national intersectoral coordination, surveillance of AMR and antimicrobial drug use, improved infection control, increased awareness of antimicrobial use and resistance, and AMR related to food-animal production. Adopted by the 2011 Regional Committee, the strategic action plan will be implemented in partnership with Member States and a broad coalition of partners, including ECDC, the European Food Safety Authority (EFSA), the United States Centers for Disease Control and Prevention (CDC), the European Society of Clinical Microbiology and Infectious Diseases (ESCMID), the Netherlands National Institute for Public Health and the Environment (RIVM), the Trans-Atlantic Task Force on Antimicrobial Resistance (TATFAR) and several WHO collaborating centres.

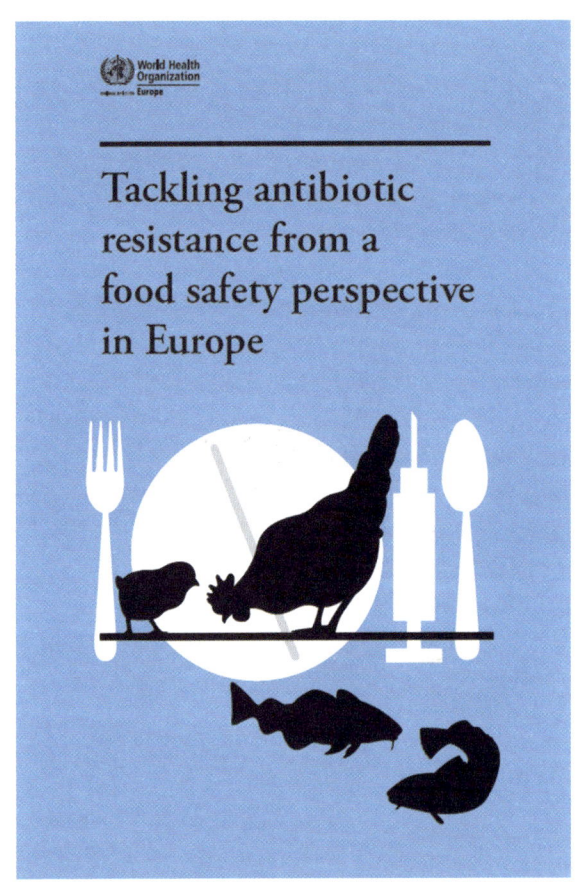

NONCOMMUNICABLE DISEASES

In 2010–2011 the Regional Office both shaped European responses to the epidemic of noncommunicable diseases (NCDs) and contributed to global initiatives.

Among the six WHO regions, NCDs affect Europe most. Together, the major NCDs – diabetes, cardiovascular diseases, cancer, chronic respiratory diseases and mental disorders – account for an estimated 86% of deaths and 77% of the disease burden in the Region. NCDs are linked by common risk factors, underlying determinants and opportunities for intervention: high blood pressure, harmful use of alcohol, tobacco use, high blood cholesterol, overweight, unhealthy diets and physical inactivity. This section gives examples of work on several of these risk factors.

European action plan shaped in a global context

In November 2010 WHO, the United Nations Economic Commission for Europe (UNECE) and the United Nations Department of Economic and Social Affairs (UNDESA) co-sponsored a high-level consultation on NCD prevention and control in the European Region, held in Oslo, Norway and hosted by the Norwegian ministries of foreign affairs and of health and care services. The Regional Office also organized an informal meeting of European countries attending the First Global Ministerial Conference on Healthy Lifestyles and Noncommunicable Disease Control (held in April 2011 and organized jointly by the Russian Federation and WHO); at this meeting, Member States decided that the summary report

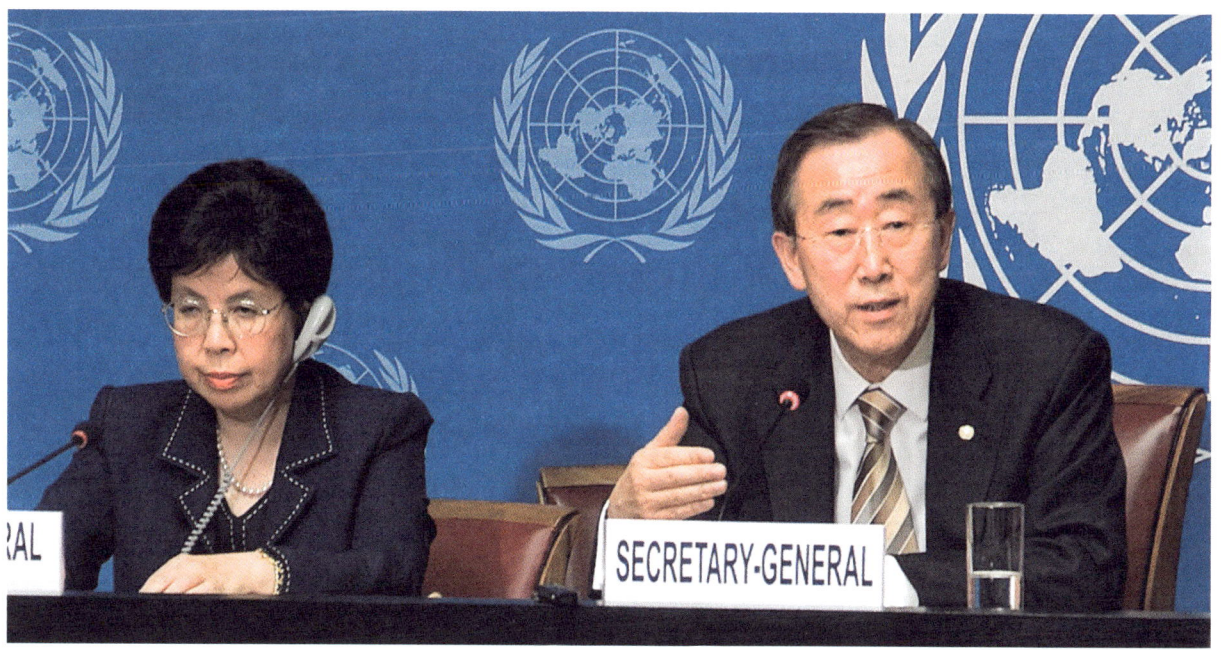

on the regional consultation *(68)* would be the Region's contribution to the United Nations General Assembly high-level meeting on NCDs in September 2011. In turn, the European response to the NCD epidemic was in line with the Political Declaration adopted by the General Assembly *(69)*.

To help shape a European response to the NCD epidemic, the Regional Office developed an action plan to implement the European strategy for NCD prevention and control *(11,70)* in 2012–2016. The Regional Office worked closely with Member States during the development process: a steering group and national focal points were appointed in January 2011; steering group members and representatives of Member States drafted the plan in February 2011, and consultation took place through a web-based process and at SCRC sessions, the European Health Policy Forum and a meeting of focal points at the Regional Office in March 2011, as well as at the Global Ministerial Conference in April.

The 2011 Regional Committee endorsed the Action Plan *(11)*. The Regional Office saw follow-up to both the Action Plan and the Political Declaration as covering three main areas: developing a comprehensive monitoring framework, working out options for effective partnerships to take multisectoral action and strengthening national policies and plans for NCD prevention and control.

Alcohol

The Regional Office followed a similar process in developing a European action plan to implement regional and global strategies on alcohol; the 2011 Regional Committee endorsed the European action plan to reduce the harmful use of alcohol 2012–2020 *(12)*. It is based on previous European strategies for 1992–2005 and is a regional iteration of WHO's global strategy to reduce harmful use of alcohol *(71)*. The Regional Office sent drafts to countries, organizations and WHO collaborating centres for comment; a consultation was held in Rome in mid-December 2010 and a global policy meeting in February 2011. For the final consultation event, the Regional Office organized a meeting of national experts on alcohol policy in Zurich, Switzerland in May 2011, in cooperation with the Alcohol Public Health Research Alliance (AMPHORA) group of alcohol experts and with the support of the Alcohol Section of the Public Health Directorate of the Federal Department of Home Affairs of Switzerland. The action plan *(12)* provides information on the harmful use of alcohol and proposes many evidence-based options for action.

Alcohol intake in the WHO European Region is the highest in the world and results in serious harm to health. In 2011, the Regional Office published a popular report giving the latest data on alcohol

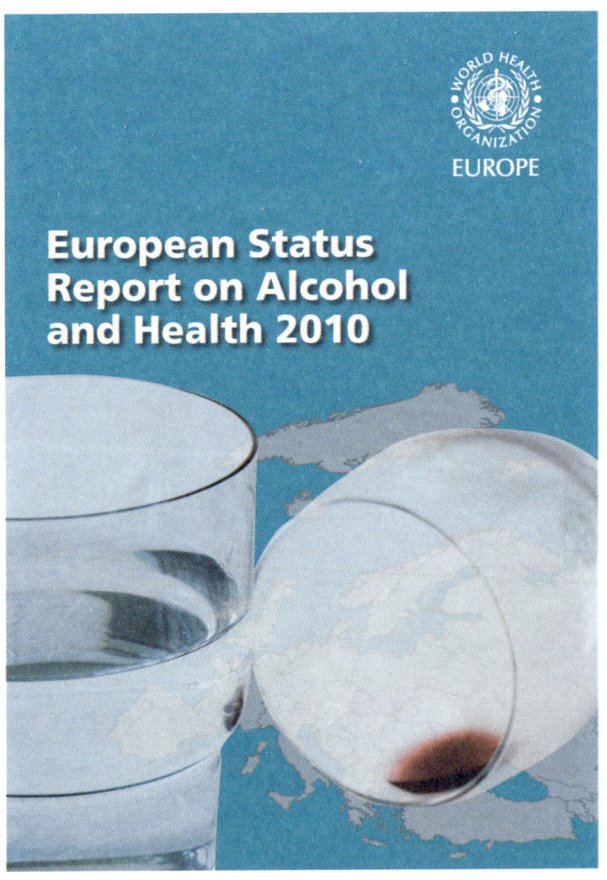

consumption and harm, and describing European countries' responses and the WHO instruments and activities to support countries *(72)*.

Tobacco control

In its work for tobacco control, the Regional Office welcomed country initiatives, such as the passage of smoke-free legislation in Hungary and Spain and its strengthening in Uzbekistan; the consideration or use of pictorial health warnings on tobacco packaging in Kazakhstan, Malta, the Russian Federation and Ukraine; and Turkmenistan's ratification of the WHO Framework Convention on Tobacco Control (FCTC) *(73)*. It supported such work by, for example, publishing a book on combating tobacco-industry marketing to women *(74)* and holding a video competition on the benefits of laws banning smoking.

To support implementation of the WHO FCTC in 2011, it organized a workshop in the Republic of Moldova attended by representatives of 47 Member States, and began preparing case studies on countries' efforts. The FCTC was the theme for World Tobacco Day 2011, on 31 May, and the Director-General's special recognition award was given to the Prime Minister of Greece, for the leadership and political commitment of the Prime Minister and the Government in taking a whole-of-government approach to tobacco control *(75)*. In 2010, the special recognition award was given to the Prime Minister of Turkey, Mr Recep Tayyip Erdogan, for his strong and continuous leadership in tobacco control.

In addition, four European countries (Poland, the Russian Federation, Turkey and Ukraine) participated in the WHO Global Adult Tobacco Survey (GATS) in 2010; three (Greece, Romania and Turkey) participated in GATS' second phase in 2011.

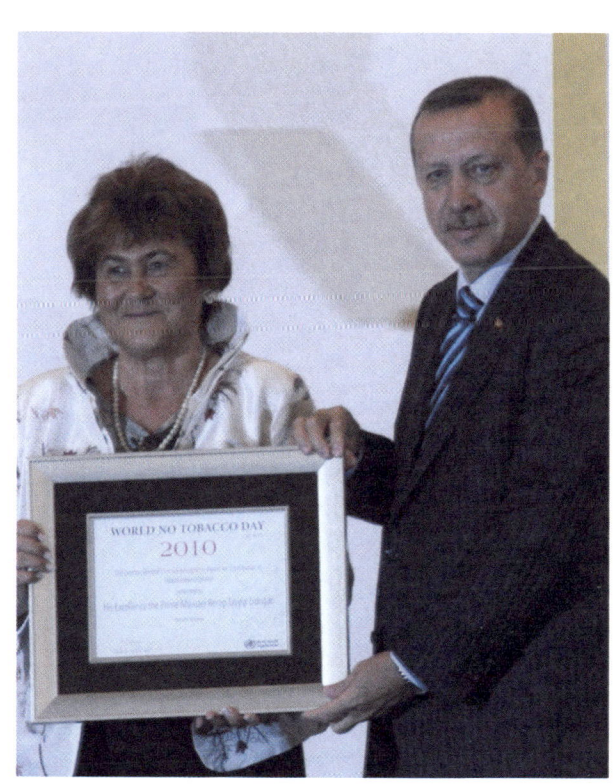

Nutrition

Information was an important focus of the Regional Office's work on nutrition. Its European Childhood Obesity Surveillance Initiative (COSI) established a standardized European surveillance system expanded to include 17 countries in 2010–2011: Belgium (Flemish region), Bulgaria, Cyprus, the Czech Republic, Greece, Hungary, Ireland, Italy, Latvia, Lithuania, Malta, Norway, Portugal, Slovenia, Spain, Sweden and the former Yugoslav Republic of Macedonia. This tool is already one of the most powerful obesity surveillance mechanisms in the world. Preliminary results indicated that, on average, 24% of children aged 6–9 years are overweight or obese *(76)*. In May 2011, the Regional Office unveiled the WHO European database on nutrition, obesity and physical activity (NOPA) *(77)*. Created in collaboration with health ministries and with support from the EC, it includes details of more than 300 national and subnational policies in the European Region.

To support implementation of the WHO European Action Plan for Food and Nutrition Policy 2007–2012 *(78)*, the Regional Office worked with its six action networks, consisting of and led by countries committed to implementing specific action. For example, the network on reducing salt in the diet met in London, United Kingdom in October 2011 to discuss policy on salt and iodine.

Mental health

In working to improve mental health, the Regional Office pursued a strategic approach, working to support Member States in providing comprehensive and community-based services. In October 2010, it organized the WHO European Conference: Better Health, Better Lives: Children and Young People with Intellectual Disabilities and Their Families in Bucharest, Romania. Health policy-makers from the 53 countries in the Region signed a declaration with an action plan *(79)* expressing their commitment to improving the lives of such young people by improving their access to high-quality health care. The declaration was supported by UNICEF, the EC, representatives of intellectually disabled young people and their families, providers of social and education services, and NGOs. The 2011 Regional Committee endorsed both declaration and action plan *(4)*.

In view of the significant gap in treatment for mental disorders, and the wide diversity of service provision, the Regional Office started work to develop a new strategy on mental health at the end of 2011. Building on the 2005 declaration and action plan for Europe *(80)*, the strategy would aim to improve the mental well-being of the population, respect the rights of people with mental health problems

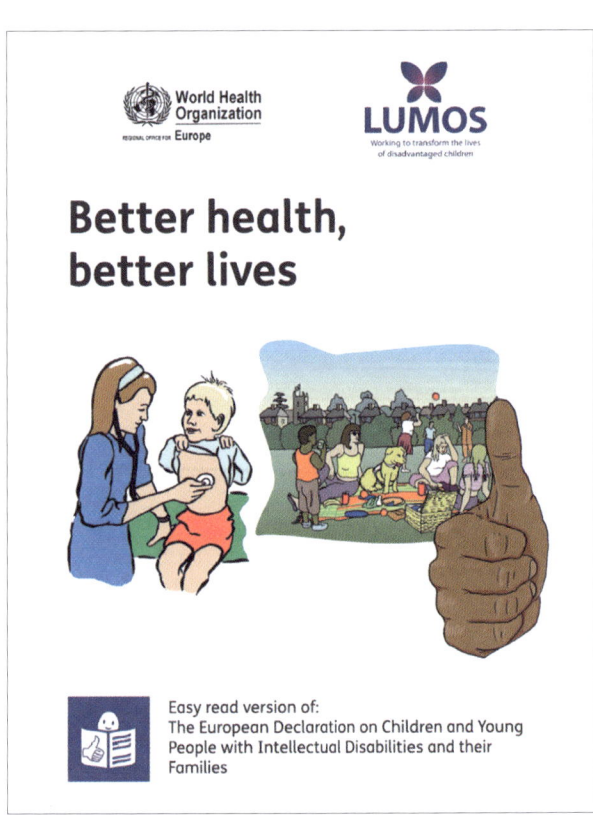

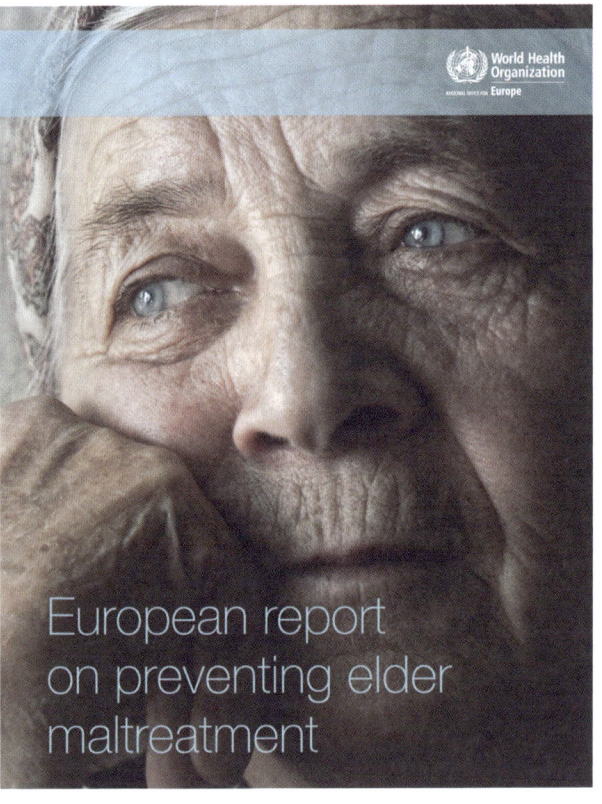

and establish accessible, safe and effective services. Extensive consultation was proposed for a two-year period leading up to the 2013 Regional Committee.

Injuries

In 2010–2011, the Regional Office's work on injuries continued to focus on prevention, supported by major publications describing not only the situation in the European Region but also options for effective policy and intervention.

For example, with EC funds, the Regional Office developed resources and tools to support national focal people across the Region and to strengthen health systems' capacity to develop national action plans and policies, monitor their implementation and report on activities. The project also facilitated the sharing of experiences in developing national action plans, advocacy and surveillance, and built capacity and mentoring in these areas through workshops held for northern and for central and southern European countries. The Regional Office presented the results in March 2010 to members of the European Parliament, WHO and EC staff, country representatives, focal people and NGOs (81).

The Regional Office recognizes the strong links between interpersonal violence and socioeconomic conditions, particularly low income at both the national level and in groups within countries. Its work therefore included publishing successful books on preventing violence towards two vulnerable groups: young and elderly people (82,83). The books took similar approaches, highlighting the biological, social, cultural, economic and environmental factors that influence the risk of being a victim or perpetrator; the protective factors that can help prevent violence; and the evidence for the efficacy

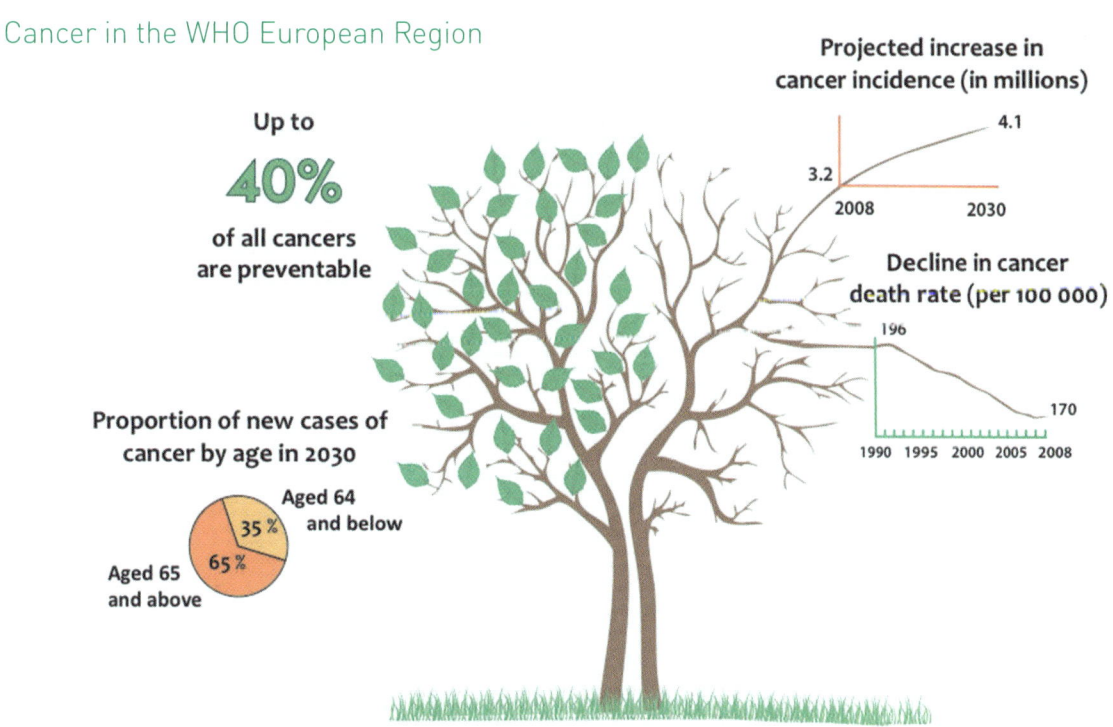

Cancer in the WHO European Region

of preventive action. Preventing injury is also an important part of the Regional Office's work for road safety (see below).

Patient, citizen and community empowerment

Patient, citizen and community empowerment were major themes in all these areas (as well as in strengthening health systems – see below). Given the influence of the common risk factors and the chronic nature of NCDs, the Regional Office led and supported initiatives to empower citizens and patients by supplying information and tools to prevent and manage these diseases. Activities included developing a background document on patient empowerment, participating in events such as the Careum Congress in Zurich, Switzerland in November 2010 and working with the Danish Ministry for the Interior and Health to prepare the first European conference on patient empowerment, to be held in April 2012 during the Danish EU Presidency.

Support to country-based activities on individual diseases

The Regional Office also supported country-based activities to tackle individual diseases such as cancer. For example, it carried out a joint mission with the International Agency for Research on Cancer (IARC) to help establish evidence-based screening programmes for breast and cervical cancer in Belarus. In addition, the Regional Office supported EU-led efforts to foster better cancer control through the European Partnership Action Against Cancer, and to promote policy attention to diabetes through participation in the EU Diabetes Working Group, held under the auspices of the Belgian EU Presidency.

HEALTH PROMOTION THROUGHOUT THE LIFE-COURSE

While working to promote health in 2010–2011, the WHO Regional Office for Europe tailored its activities to the different circumstances, issues and needs of each stage of life. This work included efforts to help countries make progress towards achieving MDGs 3–5 (on gender equality, child mortality and maternal health).

Maternal and perinatal health

Within the framework of the global WHO programme Making Pregnancy Safer, the Regional Office deploys several tools to improve the quality of maternal and neonatal care and thus reduce levels of and inequalities in morbidity and mortality. For example, Beyond the Numbers provides approaches to examining reasons behind maternal deaths and complications, such as confidential enquiry into maternal deaths and near-miss case review. The Regional Office introduced it in 14 European countries, and pilot-tested and rolled it out in 10, with the assistance of the United Nations Population Fund (UNFPA), UNICEF, GIZ (Deutsche Gesellschaft für Internationale Zusammenarbeit) and USAID. The partners and participating countries assessed their progress in introducing and using the tool at a meeting in Uzbekistan in 2010 *(84)*. In addition, the Regional Office built on earlier experience to issue an updated training package on effective perinatal care for midwives, obstetricians/gynaecologists, neonatologists and paediatric nurses in the European Region, with the assistance of John Snow Inc. and USAID *(85)*. Further, it published a description of successes in making pregnancy safer in the Region *(86)*.

In addition, with co-financing from the EU, the Regional Office completed a project in Kazakhstan in 2011. Its aim was to improve the quality of care for pregnant women, mothers, newborn babies and children by introducing evidence-based care and thus to assist Kazakhstan in achieving MDGs 4 and 5. A publication describes the project's successes from the viewpoints of doctors, midwives and service users *(87)*.

The Regional Office's work to prevent cervical cancer is discussed above.

Childhood and adolescence

Providing information as a basis for policy-making is a vital part of the Regional Office's work for young people's health. In 2011, the Regional Office issued eight publications in a series calling for a whole-of-society response to the gender differences and inequalities that affect illness, health and well-being

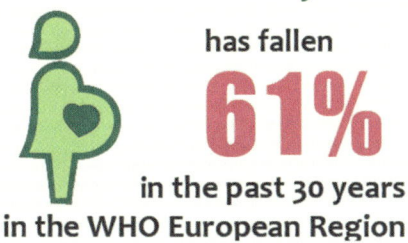

The **maternal mortality ratio** has fallen **61%** in the past 30 years in the WHO European Region

in girls and boys in the European Region. They describe the evidence for gender-responsive action to promote health and well-being; to prevent and manage overweight and obesity, HIV/AIDS and sexually transmitted infections, adolescent pregnancy, chronic conditions, injuries and substance abuse; and to prevent violence *(88)*. The aim is to supply a useful tool to help transform evidence into action and to strengthen innovative ways of working across sectors, one of the core policy actions of Health 2020 *(5)*.

Similarly, towards the end of 2011, the Regional Office prepared the latest international report on the Health Behaviour in School-aged Children (HBSC) study *(89)*. The aim was to provide a rigorous, systematic statistical base for describing cross-national patterns, in terms of the magnitude and direction of differences between subgroups of young people aged 11, 13 and 15 years, thus contributing to a better understanding of the social determinants of health and well-being among young people, and providing the means to help protect and promote their health. The 2009/2010 survey covered 43 countries and regions in the WHO European Region and North America, and addressed young people's social context (relations with family, peers and school), physical health and satisfaction with life, health behaviours (patterns of eating, tooth brushing and physical activity) and risk behaviours (use of tobacco, alcohol and cannabis, sexual behaviour, fighting and bullying).

As in other areas of work, the Regional Office supported country initiatives to protect and promote young people's health, often specified in BCAs. For example, it supported the Republic of Moldova and Ukraine in reorganizing their school health services, by holding workshops on monitoring and evaluating these services and building the competencies of their personnel, in early 2011. It also published the results of a survey on improving hospital care for children in Armenia, Kazakhstan, Turkmenistan and Uzbekistan *(90)*.

Sexual and reproductive health

With partners including the EU, the Regional Office supported the introduction of integrated, evidence-based care to improve sexual and reproductive health in its work with countries, often through BCAs and with the involvement of country offices. For example, it assisted Armenia, Azerbaijan, Georgia, Kyrgyzstan, Tajikistan and Turkey in improving the quality of family planning services in primary health care. In 2010 in Kaunas, Lithuania, the Regional Office held its third course to build capacity in operations research on reproductive health; 20 programme managers and researchers from Albania, Latvia, Romania, Serbia and Turkey analysed the situation in their countries and discussed the priority areas for operational research with the national counterparts in their health ministries.

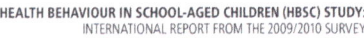
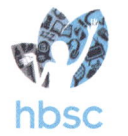

In 2010, the Regional Office and the Federal Centre for Health Education (BZgA) published standards for sexuality education in Europe with step-by-step instructions and a detailed matrix to support health and education professionals in their efforts to guarantee children accurate and sensitively presented information about sexuality *(91)*. Then the partners held a consultation at which representatives of ministries of health and education and of civil-society organizations discussed ways to promote and use the standards to improve sexuality education in their countries.

In 2011, with funds from UNFPA, the Regional Office published two issues of *Entre Nous*, the European magazine for sexual and reproductive health *(92)*. They focused on the progress made in sexual health across Europe; its role in overall health, well-being and the quality of life; the different needs of adolescents, older people, migrants, people living with HIV and people with disabilities; and the relationship between health inequities, the social determinants of health and sexual and reproductive health.

Active and healthy ageing

In 2011, the Regional Office started to develop a strategy and action plan on healthy ageing in Europe, and completed the first draft. The strategy will have four components: healthy ageing over the life-course, supportive environments, strengthening health systems for ageing populations and addressing the gaps in research and evidence. As with the European Action Plan on NCDs *(11)*, the Regional Office used a set of criteria to select a limited number of priority interventions (such as prevention of falls, vaccination of older people and improved training of staff) and supportive interventions (prevention of elder maltreatment and social isolation, and development of strategies for ensuring the quality of care for older people). Wide consultation – at a meeting for national focal points, with the SCRC and through the Internet – was planned to refine the draft for submission to the Regional Committee in 2012. As mentioned, the Regional Office also published an important book on preventing elder maltreatment *(83)*.

MDGs

In 2010, the Regional Office identified the United Nations MDGs as a cross-Office priority, paying attention to reinforcing synergies in concerted and coordinated action to reach them, to strengthen health systems and to address other health challenges in the Region such as NCDs. The Regional Director appointed a special representative on the MDGs.

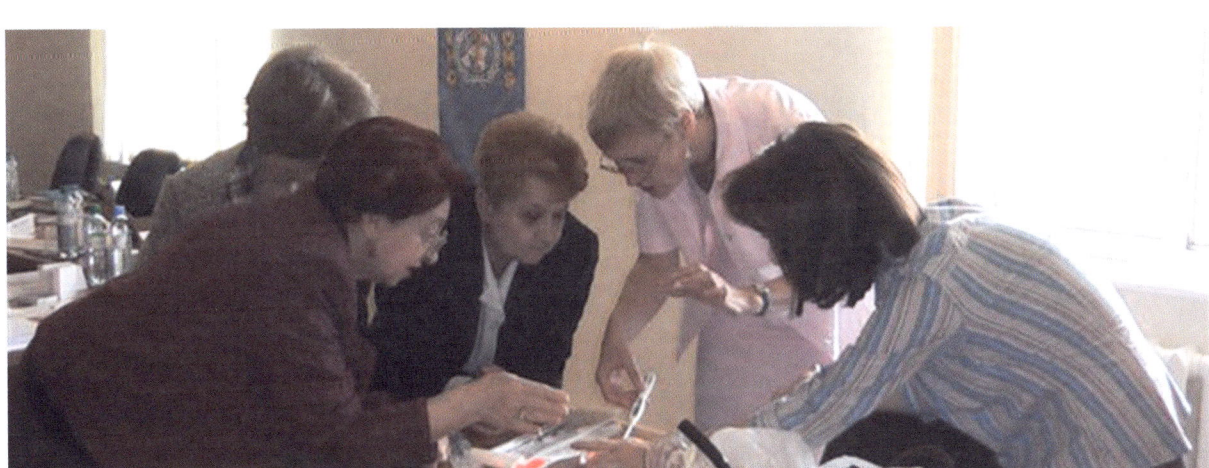

In late 2010, WHO held a meeting in Durres, Albania to review progress towards achieving MDGs 3–5. The participants – national focal points for family and community health and government officials from more than 25 countries, and representatives of United Nations agencies and other partners – drew conclusions on a range of actions needed *(93)*. The Regional Office contributed to high-level events organized by Member States: a forum for eastern Europe and central Asia on MDG 6, and international forums on MDGs 4 and 5 hosted by the Russian Federation and Uzbekistan in late 2011. In addition, the Regional Office published its biennial report on progress towards MDGs 4–6 in 2011, including policy considerations for accelerating progress towards each *(94)*.

In line with Health 2020 *(5)*, the new European health policy, and under the umbrella of the Regional Coordination Mechanism (RCM), the Regional Office played an active role by leading an interagency working group of United Nations agencies on tackling inequities in progress towards MDGs. The working group held its first meeting in December 2010, and was endorsed during the RCM meeting in March 2011.

In this context, WHO provided input to a technical meeting on reducing health inequalities in eastern Europe and central Asia, with a focus on vulnerable groups and sexual and reproductive health, convened by UNFPA in Turkey in March 2011. Its outcomes included agreement to move forward with an interagency proposal for 2012–2015 on "scaling up action on MDGs 4 and 5 in the context of the Decade for Roma Inclusion". WHO led work on drafting this interagency proposal. Other working-group products agreed for 2011 included an interagency report on progress towards the MDGs in the European Region; cooperation on events and advocacy, communication and capacity-building activities; and exploration of opportunities for joint country work.

In addition, the Regional Office worked with WHO headquarters to conduct the WHO/UNICEF Joint Monitoring Programme for Water Supply and Sanitation, which monitors progress towards achieving MDG 7; target 7.C aims to halve, by 2015, the proportion of people without sustainable access to safe drinking-water and basic sanitation.

Ottawa Charter for Health Promotion

A ceremony at the 2011 session of the Regional Committee commemorated the twenty-fifth anniversary of the signing of the Ottawa Charter for Health Promotion, and celebrated the change in public health that the Charter helped to accomplish *(4,95)*.

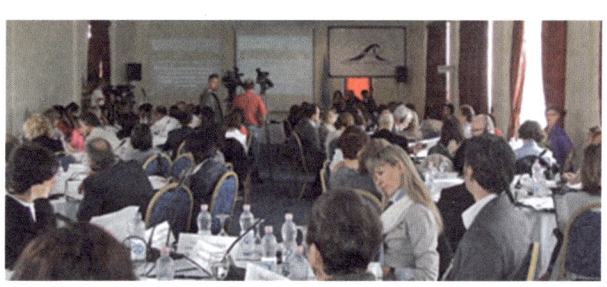

STRENGTHENING OF HEALTH SYSTEMS

In 2010–2011, the Regional Office continued to help countries strengthen and reform their health systems through such means as tailored individual support (often delivered through BCAs), support to countries' implementation of the Tallinn Charter and achievement of universal coverage, the creation of a framework to strengthen public health capacities and services in Europe and work to strengthen health personnel. While important in itself, strengthening people-centred health systems and public health capacities is also essential to implementing Health 2020.

Strengthening of health systems

To support countries in implementing the Tallinn Charter: "Health Systems for Health and Wealth" *(28)* and to gauge its effectiveness, the Regional Office held two expert consultations in October 2010 and January 2011 and set up a working group, consisting of representatives of nine Member States, to compile an interim report on implementation of the Charter. The Regional Office presented the report to the Regional Committee at its 2011 session *(96)*. It draws on a wealth of information in the replies to a questionnaire sent to all Member States in the Region.

Meeting in Andorra, the European Health Policy Forum confirmed that the Tallinn Charter, particularly its focus on monitoring and evaluation, had led to a more vigorous policy dialogue on the importance of preserving, reforming and investing in health systems, and that countries were putting its values and policy objectives into practice. The

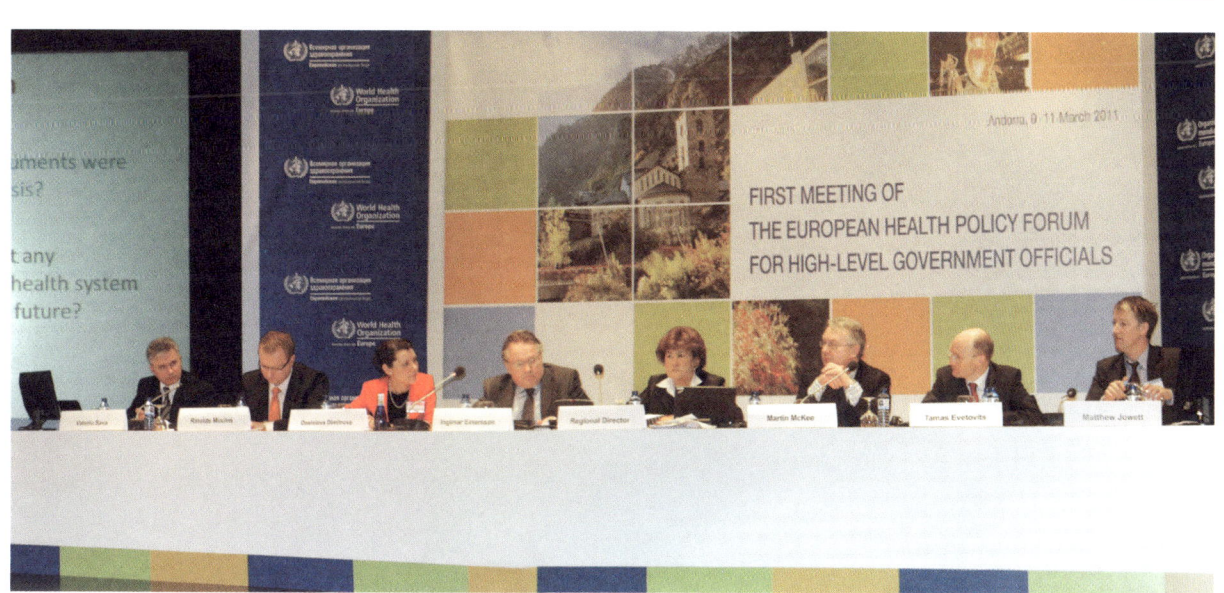

Health 2020 policy framework will be informed by the lessons learned. Along with the interim report, the Regional Office presented to the 2011 Regional Committee a consolidated package of the strategies and services that it can offer to strengthen health systems *(97)*.

The Regional Office also developed a new approach that applies the health systems approach, or systems thinking, to diseases and conditions such as NCDs and M/XDR-TB. This fresh approach came from 15 years of generic work to strengthen health systems, putting the building blocks in place to ensure health systems' strategic orientation towards health outcomes. It requires putting service delivery in the centre and has three pillars:

- starting with expected health outcomes and priorities;
- focusing on optimal service delivery strategies, in which the content comes from technical areas; and
- identifying barriers that prevent health systems from providing effective services, which can be grouped under the headings of service delivery, governance, financing and resources.

The changes in the European and global health contexts, the pressures exerted by the financial crisis, the rise in NCDs and other challenges highlight the need for comprehensive system responses. Against this background, the WHO Global Policy Group led a project on national health policy frameworks with system-wide analysis.

Supporting universal coverage and minimizing the effects of the financial crisis

To pursue equity in health, the Regional Office supports countries in their efforts to build health systems providing universal coverage to the population, and to minimize the harmful effects of the financial crisis. Training to build capacity in countries was a particularly important tool in this area in 2010–2011. For example, the Regional Office:

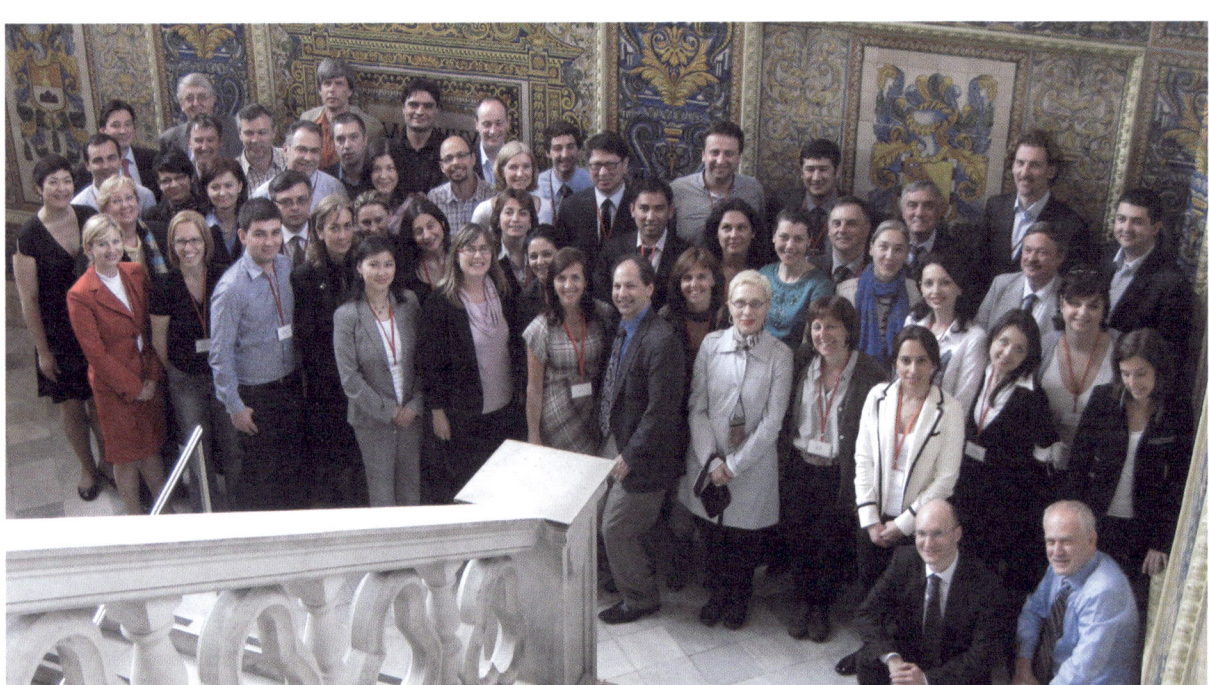

- with the Ministry of Social Affairs of Estonia and the Estonian Health Insurance Fund, and financial support from the European Social Fund, coordinated two flagship courses on health system strengthening and sustainable financing in October 2010 and April 2011, for over 60 government and health insurance fund officials, and other health-sector stakeholders from Estonia, Latvia, Lithuania and Poland;
- with the World Bank Institute and the Health Policy Analysis Centre in Kyrgyzstan, held the seventh annual flagship course on strengthening health systems through improved health financing and service delivery in November 2010 in Barcelona, Spain, for 47 health professionals from Armenia, Azerbaijan, Kazakhstan, Kyrgyzstan, the Republic of Moldova, Tajikistan, Turkmenistan and Uzbekistan; and
- started a new course in Barcelona in May 2011, focusing on how to improve health system performance through better health financing policy, and specifically on universal coverage.

The Regional Office published three papers in 2010 on health financing and population coverage in Estonia and the Republic of Moldova *(98)*, and Regional Office staff made a major contribution to *The world health report 2010. Health systems financing: the path to universal coverage (99)*.

Action plan to strengthen public health

The Regional Office worked on a framework of action to strengthen public health capacities and services in Europe, complementary to Health 2020, for completion in 2012. It based the development process on both research and wide consultation, and launched an evaluation of public health services in selected western European countries and a study on policy tools and instruments for public health. In developing and revising the document, the Regional Office held a small expert meeting in November 2010 and consultation meetings with public health experts in January and April 2011, as well as presenting it to the European Health Policy Forum for review. The Forum fully supported the action framework. Later in 2011, the Regional Office consulted with Member States at the SEEHN Health Ministers' Forum (see above), conferences held by ASPHER and the holder of the EU Presidency, its first consultation on human resources for public health in October and the Health 2020 conference.

The draft European Action Plan for Strengthening Public Health Capacities and Services *(100,101)* lists 10 essential public health operations (EPHOs) that were pilot-tested in the European Region for four years, sets out a framework for action and outlines the role of the Regional Office. The revised EPHO tool – a web-based instrument for self-assessment of public health services – was planned to be tested in a number of countries.

Recognizing the Regional Office's contribution to public health, ASPHER awarded the Andrija Štampar Medal to the Regional Director in 2011.

Support to health personnel

The Regional Office promoted the WHO Global Code of Practice on the International Recruitment of Health Personnel *(102)*, for example, at the Subregional Policy Dialogue on Health Professional Mobility in Central and Eastern Europe in April 2011, organized by the Government of Hungary as the country holding the EU Presidency. The European Observatory on Health Systems and Policies presented a study at the event, on an EU project on professional mobility and health systems in 17 European countries. Also in April, the Regional Office invited Member States and other stakeholders to contribute to the web-based public hearing on the draft guidelines for monitoring implementation of the Global Code.

In 2010–2011, the Regional Office worked to strengthen its cooperation with associations of health professionals through annual meetings and joint projects with the European Forum of Medical Associations (EFMA) and the European Forum of National Nursing and Midwifery Associations (EFNNMA). With the support of the Polish Presidency of the EU, the Regional Office took part in meetings of countries' chief medical and chief nursing officers in October 2011, to revitalize cooperation with these networks. In addition, with the support of the Hungarian EU Presidency, the Hungarian Ministry of National Resources, the Europharm Forum, the WHO Regional Office for Europe and the Hungarian National Committee of Pharmaceutical Care held a conference for decision-makers on pharmacists' contribution to public health in NCDs in June 2011.

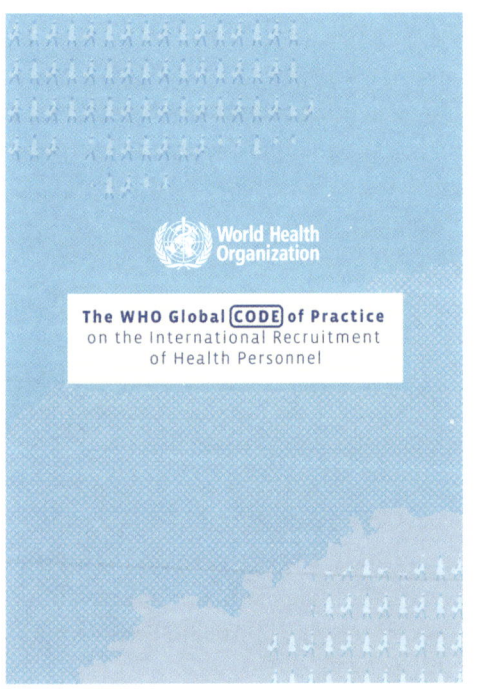

Patient empowerment

Patient empowerment is as vital to strong health systems as to the struggle against NCDs (see above). Through BCAs, the Regional Office supported a range of work for patient safety and the quality of care. These included:

- pilot-testing patient-safety tools in Albania and Serbia;
- studies on ways to improve patients' health literacy and the capacity to reduce safety risks through hand hygiene (Bulgaria) and in blood transfusion (France), prescriptions in primary care (Poland) and elective surgery (Portugal); and
- round-table discussions to explore reporting systems for adverse events in the Czech Republic, Slovakia and Slovenia (103).

With partners, the Regional Office sought to build capacity: for health promotion in hospitals in the Czech Republic, and in safe clinical transfusion practice in Albania, curricula on patient safety in Romania, research on patient safety in Slovenia, and hand hygiene and prevention of nosocomial infections in Uzbekistan.

Information

Finally, the Regional Office provided valuable information on health systems. For example, the Observatory issued profiles of the health systems of seven countries in 2010, and of seven more (Kyrgyzstan, Poland, Portugal, the Russian Federation, Slovakia, Turkey and the United Kingdom (England)) in 2011 (104), along with a study of cross-border health care in the EU (105).

ENVIRONMENT AND HEALTH

In 2010–2011, the Regional Office continued working with countries and partners on a wide range of environment and health issues. Examples of its work in 2010–2011 include publishing important information that countries could use to take action and supporting countries in taking the next steps in the European environment and health process.

Next steps in the European environment and health process

Fifth Ministerial Conference on Environment and Health

The Regional Office organized the Fifth Ministerial Conference on Environment and Health, hosted by Italy and held on 10–12 March 2010 in Parma, as the latest milestone in the European environment and health process, then in its twentieth year. Focused on protecting children's health in a changing environment, the Conference set Europe's agenda on emerging environmental health challenges for the years to come *(106)*. The participants adopted the Parma Declaration, the first time-bound outcome of the environment and health process. In it, the 53 Member States in the Region set clear targets to reduce the harm to health from environmental threats in the next decade, agreeing to implement national programmes to provide equal opportunities to each child by 2020 by ensuring access to safe water and sanitation, opportunities for physical activity and a healthy diet, improved air quality and an environment free of toxic chemicals.

The other main Conference outcomes were a regional framework for action to protect health in an environment challenged by climate change, and a new institutional framework to strengthen and guide the process until the next conference, planned for 2016: the European Environment and Health

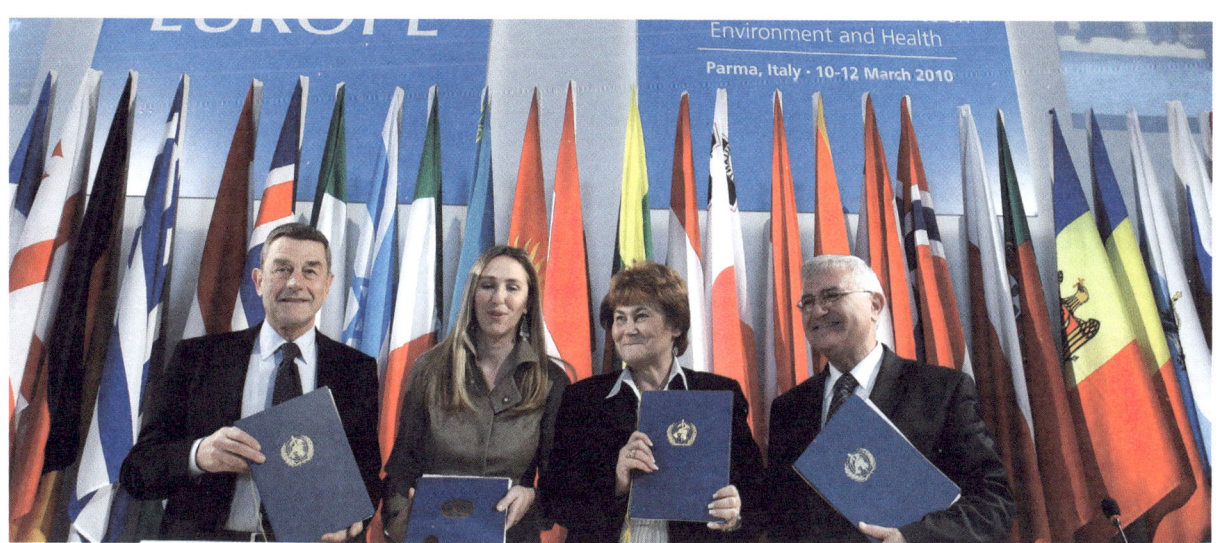

Ministerial Board (the driving force of international policies on environment and health) and the European Environment and Health Task Force (the leading international intersectoral body for implementation and monitoring). Both report to WHO and the United Nations Economic Commission for Europe (UNECE). In September 2010, the Regional Committee endorsed the outcomes of the Conference *(3)*.

Following the Conference, the Regional Office provided technical and policy support to Albania, Croatia, Montenegro, Serbia and Turkey in implementing WHO's global plan of action on workers' health 2008–2017. This resulted in the implementation of national strategies and action plans on occupational health services, capacity building and integration of occupational health services into primary health care. The Regional Office also provided technical and policy support in developing national programmes for elimination of asbestos-related diseases.

New course for environment and health governance

Meeting for the first time in Paris, France in May 2011, the Ministerial Board agreed on how to monitor progress in reducing the adverse health impact of environmental threats across the WHO European Region. The Regional Committee had appointed the health ministers of France, Malta, Serbia and Slovenia, and the UNECE Committee on Environmental Policy had appointed the environment ministers of Azerbaijan, Belarus, Romania and Turkey to the Board for 2011–2012. Other members included the WHO Regional Director for Europe, the Executive Secretary of UNECE, the Director of the United Nations Environment Programme (UNEP) Regional Office for Europe and the EC.

The Task Force met for the first time in Bled, Slovenia in October 2011 *(107)*. Members reviewed and discussed developments since the Parma Conference and proposed areas of joint action, including policy, the evidence base, international commitments and emerging issues related to energy and health, intersectoral work, sustainable development, prevention of NCDs and inequalities, climate change, water, sanitation and asbestos. Members stressed the importance of developing a strong communication strategy and decided to strengthen their collaboration, particularly on developing indicators for reporting progress towards the Parma commitments.

Environmental determinants of health

One citizen out of five in the WHO European Region dies from environment-associated diseases. Improving the natural and man-made environments could save nearly 1.8 million lives every year. The environmental burden of ill health varies significantly across the Region, ranging from 14% to 54%. In all countries, the poor are at much greater risk.

In 2010–2011, the Regional Office's work on environment and health covered a wide range of topics, notably climate change, food safety and safe water and sanitation; and included assessment of health risks of major environmental factors, such as air and noise pollution, and inadequate housing and radiation. Information was a vital tool in this work; for example, the Environment and Health Information System (ENHIS) provided the basis for reporting on the situation and trends to the Parma Conference *(108)*. In addition, publications on environmental determinants of health remained among the Regional Office's most popular products. For example, as part of a global process, the Regional Office published WHO guidelines for the protection of public health from a number of dangerous chemicals commonly present in indoor air in December 2010 *(109)*; they provide a scientific basis for legally enforceable standards. In 2011, the Regional Office published the first report assessing the burden of disease from environmental noise in Europe *(110)* and that associated with inadequate housing *(111)*.

Environment and health

In 2010–2011, the Regional Office worked with WHO headquarters on an assessment of water supply and sanitation that revealed decreasing access to piped water in central Asia. With partners, the Regional Office provided training on water-safety planning in Albania, Georgia, Tajikistan, Turkmenistan and Ukraine. In addition, the Regional Office and UNECE jointly organized the Second Meeting of the Parties to the Protocol on Water and Health, which was held in November 2010 in Bucharest, Romania and hosted by the Ministry of Environment. Participants representing 33 countries and United Nations, intergovernmental and nongovernmental organizations discussed the work carried out over the previous three years (including ratification and implementation of the Protocol), approved four documents, and endorsed a new Regional Office report *(112)*, as well as welcoming the Protocol's twenty-fifth Party, Bosnia and Herzegovina.

Transport and road safety

Under the framework of the Transport, Health and Environment Pan European Programme (THE PEP), the Regional Office launched the Decade of Action for Road Safety 2011–2020 in the WHO European Region at the May 2011 summit of the International Transport Forum (ITF) in Leipzig, Germany, along with a new health economic assessment tool (HEAT) to enable countries to measure the potential economic savings from making cycling and walking safer and more popular *(113)*. In addition, many countries – including Albania, Belarus, Croatia, Hungary, the Republic of Moldova, the Russian Federation, Slovakia, Slovenia, the United Kingdom and Uzbekistan – marked the start of the Decade with launch events, meetings and other activities, often with the support of WHO country offices.

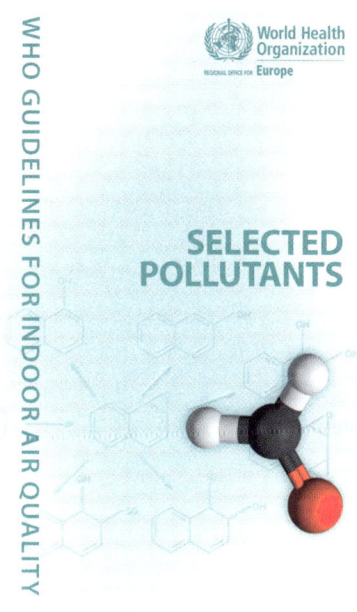

Chernobyl commemoration

Taking part in marking the twenty-fifth anniversary of the Chernobyl disaster, which affected large areas in Belarus, the Russian Federation and Ukraine, helped to renew support for the people affected and build on the lessons learnt. WHO summarized its assessments of the health effects of the accident in two landmark reports, published in 2006 and 2011 *(114)*. The WHO Regional Director for Europe joined other leaders from around the world to commemorate the accident, and to review the reconstruction and development of the affected communities, at a summit and an international conference on the safe use of nuclear energy held in Kyiv in April 2011.

PREPAREDNESS, SURVEILLANCE AND RESPONSE

In 2010–2011, the Regional Office not only helped countries cope with emergencies and public health crises but also assessed and helped them improve their preparedness and their capacity to respond.

IHR implementation and compliance

The IHR *(115)* remained a priority for the Regional Office. To support Member States in developing and strengthening their core capacities for implementation by the deadline of June 2012, activities in this area, carried out in partnership with the EU and other institutions and agencies, focused on:

- increasing awareness and political commitment at the highest level;
- endorsing the role of national IHR focal points;
- supporting the initiation of national multisectoral implementation processes and the development of national action plans;
- assisting with reporting; and
- providing guidance and training in relation to IHR implementation at ports, airports and ground crossings.

In cooperation with Member States and other partners, these priorities are reflected in events organized by the Regional Office, such as the training course and workshops held in Copenhagen in October 2010 and December 2011, and in Uzbekistan, Turkey and France in April, June and September 2011, respectively *(116)*.

Preparedness

Within the IHR framework, the Regional Office assisted countries in increasing their readiness for and ability to respond to emergencies by assessing and strengthening health systems' preparedness, offering guidance on hospital resilience and safety, and providing training and capacity building. For example, it assessed preparedness in Turkey *(117)* and Kazakhstan; and, with the EC Directorate-General for Health and Consumers, developed a toolkit to assess health-system capacity *(118)* and published a checklist for hospital emergency response to help hospital administrators and emergency managers respond effectively to the most likely disaster scenarios *(119)*. The toolkit was rolled out in 12 European countries and comprehensive assessment reports documented national health systems' emergency preparedness.

In addition, with large sporting events planned to take place in the Region in 2012 (the European football championship to be hosted by Poland and Ukraine and the Olympic Games to be hosted by the United Kingdom), the Regional Office worked with national authorities to anticipate and prepare for the associated health needs and prepared health advice for people attending the events *(120)*.

Further, WHO supported training in public health and emergency management and organized regional and national programmes to build capacity. Finally, the Regional Office published the first part of an atlas of disaster risks in the Region on CD-ROM, as part of a global series *(121)*.

Preparedness, surveillance and response

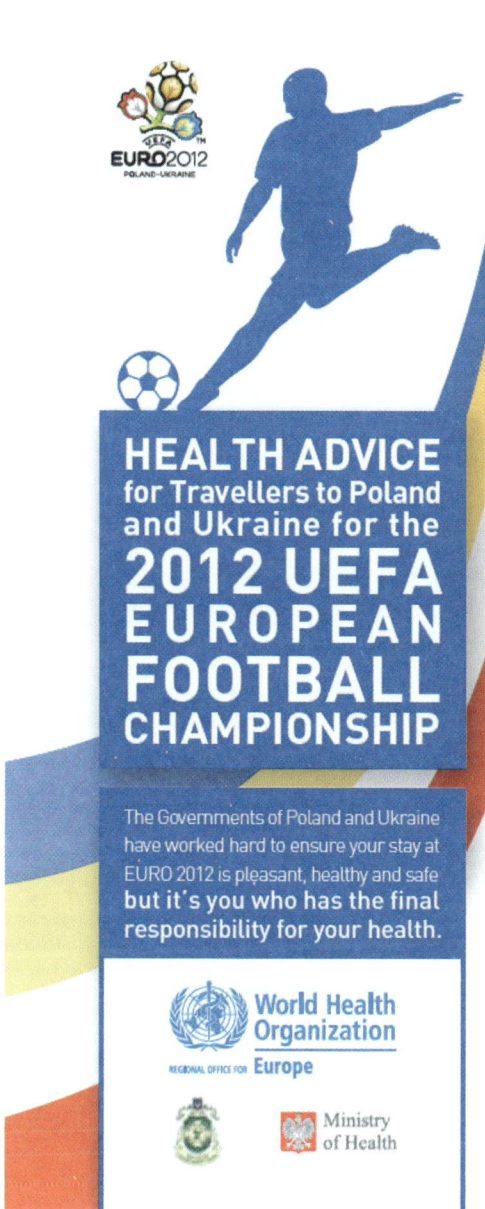

Alert and response

The Regional Office constantly monitors and screens a great variety of signals on public health events, irrespective of their nature or cause, and on natural and man-made disasters. This all-hazards event-based surveillance uses both official and unofficial sources, and takes place under the IHR framework in close collaboration with ECDC and WHO headquarters.

In 2010–2011, the Regional Office recorded and followed up over 400 signals (3–4 events per week). It took further action on 122 events (1–2 per week) that included communications with the national IHR focal point of the country concerned and risk assessment, usually involving WHO headquarters and the relevant WHO country office. In addition, the Regional Office maintained regular contact with other partners, particularly ECDC. Joint WHO–ECDC missions responded to disease outbreaks in the Region: West Nile virus in Romania and malaria in Greece.

During the biennium, the Regional Office responded to seven major environmental crises, including: the eruption of a volcano in Iceland, a severe heat-wave and wildfires in the Russian Federation, a chemical accident in Hungary (October 2010), flooding in Balkan countries in 2010, and cholera cases in Ukraine and other emergencies discussed in this report in 2011.

In the wake of civil unrest in southern Kyrgyzstan, in November 2010 WHO, its partners and the country's Ministry of Health rolled out a series of new projects to support health services and ensure access to care, particularly emergency services and mental health care. A donation of US$ 1 million from the Russian Federation made this support possible.

After people displaced by the crisis in northern Africa came to Greece, Italy and Malta, a joint mission of the Ministry of Health of Italy and the Regional Office in March 2011 called for stronger disease surveillance and prevention measures related to water and sanitation, and rigorous environmental control. The Regional Office conducted similar assessment missions in Greece and Malta, jointly with these countries' health ministries and ECDC. Recommendations included harmonizing and strengthening public health preparedness for an influx of migrants. At the 2011 World Health Assembly, Italy and the Regional Office agreed to conduct a three-year project on the public health aspects of migration.

The Ministry of Health of Italy, in collaboration with the EC Directorate-General for Health and Consumers and with the support of the WHO Regional Office for Europe, organized a meeting in Rome in April 2011, attended by high-level health officials from Cyprus, France, Greece, Malta and Spain, and representatives of the relevant United Nations and EU agencies (including ECDC), the WHO Regional Office for the Eastern Mediterranean, the Office of the United Nations High Commissioner for Refugees and the International Organization for Migration. The participants reviewed the health situation and the initiatives taken in northern Africa and in European countries and discussed how countries and agencies could prepare, coordinate and manage international support.

A food-safety emergency arose in the Region at the end of May 2011, when Germany notified WHO (under the IHR) of an outbreak of enterohaemorrhagic *Escherichia coli* (EHEC) infection, with cases of haemolytic uraemic syndrome (HUS). WHO shared information with health authorities in other countries, offered technical assistance and facilitated collaboration between laboratories to help countries without the capacity to detect the unusual *E. coli* serogroup involved, maintained close contact with relevant authorities and issued regular updates on the evolving situation *(122)*.

Earthquakes struck Van province in Turkey in October and November 2011. While the Turkish authorities carried out response activities and fully managed the rescue operations, the WHO Country Office, Turkey, within the United Nations country team, worked closely with the Ministry of Health to follow the damage assessments, and to monitor the situation and evolving health needs.

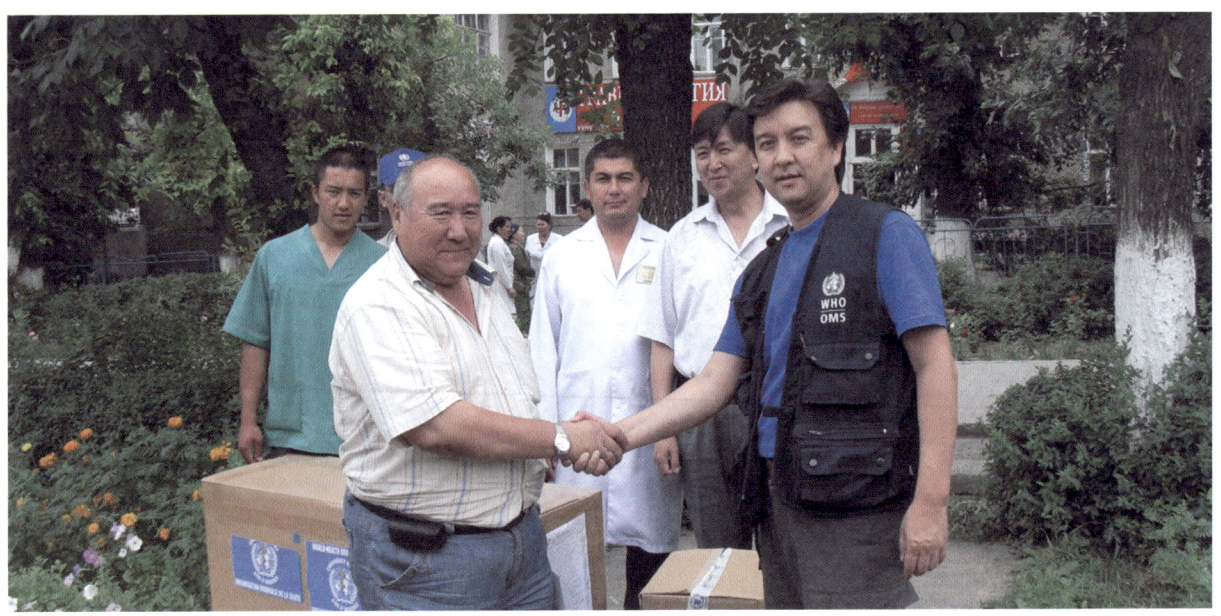

EVIDENCE AND INFORMATION AS BASIS FOR POLICY-MAKING

Providing evidence and information for policy-makers was an important part of the Regional Office's work in many areas, as preceding sections show, but the primary aim of some activities in 2010–2011.

Integrated health-information system and strategy for Europe

As mentioned, the EC and the Regional Office agreed to develop an integrated health information system for Europe as one of their six areas for intensified cooperation (*16,17*). The harmonization of health information and platforms across Europe would permit comparisons across the Region, reduce the burden on countries embarking on new health-information systems and increase consistency in the generation and dissemination of knowledge for health policy. The partners aimed to make the best possible use of already standardized quality indicators, and avoid double reporting and collection, and the use of different definitions and coding of indicators wherever possible. In 2011, the Regional Office and EC started to map their health-information work (including databases, system architectures and quality assessment), to identify how further integration or streamlining of health-information systems could be made possible and beneficial from the political, legal, and technical points of view. They invited OECD to become a partner in this task.

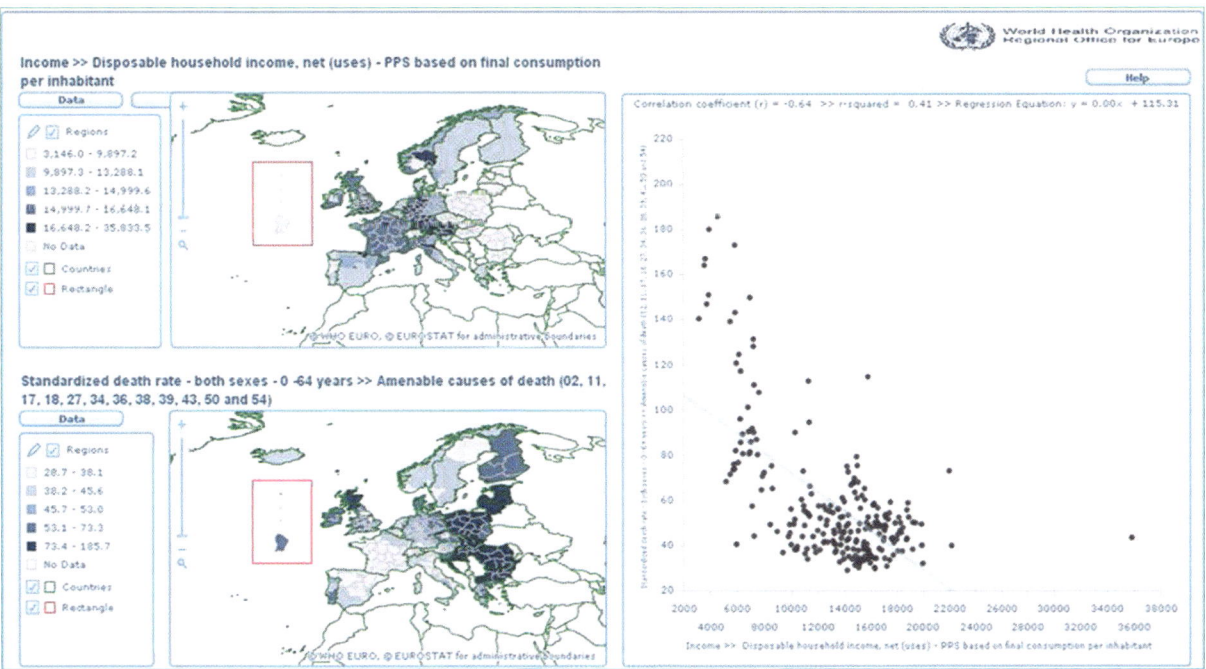

This work was part of the Regional Office's efforts to develop a strategy for health information to help reduce inequalities in health information between Member States, prevent multiplication of requests, alleviate the reporting burden and potentially lead to a joint strategy with other agencies. Work to follow the road map for the health-information system was part of this effort. The framework for the proposed strategy has four sections:

- vision, mission statement, target audience and background;
- objectives, strategic goals, outputs and expected outcomes;
- elements required for implementation, partnerships, and monitoring and evaluation; and
- conclusions, implementation plan and definitions/references.

Towards the end of 2011, the Regional Office sought the approval of the SCRC *(25)* and partners on the structure, content and feasibility of the framework, and on the implementation plan.

Tools

As part of work for greater equity in health, a multidonor project on inequalities in health-system performance and their social determinants in Europe, led by the Regional Office and the EC, made impressive progress. It started in 2007 with the objectives of mapping health inequalities in the EU and selected neighbouring countries, using a range of Eurostat indicator datasets, and developing resources to assist policy-makers in taking action. A system of interactive atlases of health inequalities in Europe was developed *(123)*, supported by a web-based resource of examples of action that health systems can take to tackle socially determined health inequalities *(124)* and a companion publication *(125)*.

The Regional Office started work on new tools for data analysis and display in 2011, aiming to complete them by the end of 2012. These tools will permit new analyses of data on an integrated database platform, and easy display of results on new data dashboards.

Publishing

In addition to the many publications mentioned above, the Regional Office published a number of products, mainly on health and health systems in the European Region, whose success testified to their usefulness. For example, the European Health for All database *(36)*, updated twice each year, remained the most widely used product in 2010–2011.

In 2010, the Regional Office published two policy summaries and three policy briefs, produced by the Health Evidence Network (HEN) and the European Observatory on Health Systems and Policies to support the EU presidencies of Spain and Belgium *(126)*. Addressing questions about health systems and health care policies in Europe, these publications aimed to provide high-quality, accessible material of immediate interest to national policy- and decision-makers seeking key messages based on solid foundations, and to researchers and experts seeking brief but authoritative reviews. Popular publications on health systems from the Observatory are discussed above *(104,105)*, but other notable products from 2010–2011 included studies on promoting innovation in antibiotic research, implementing health financing reform in countries in transition, governing public hospitals and making the case for investing in health systems *(127–130)*. Finally, the Regional Office and the Observatory began a study to make the economic case for investing in public health, health promotion and disease prevention interventions across the European Region.

REFERENCES[2]

1. *Better health for Europe: adapting the Regional Office for Europe to the changing European environment: the Regional Director's perspective.* Copenhagen, WHO Regional Office for Europe, 2010 (EUR/RC60/8; http://www.euro.who.int/en/who-we-are/governance/regional-committee-for-europe/past-sessions/sixtieth-session/documentation/working-documents/eurrc608).

2. *WHO Regional Committee for Europe resolution EUR/RC60/R2 on better health for Europe: adapting the Regional Office for Europe to the changing European environment: the Regional Director's perspective.* Copenhagen, WHO Regional Office for Europe, 2010 (http://www.euro.who.int/en/who-we-are/governance/regional-committee-for-europe/past-sessions/sixtieth-session/resolutions/eurrc60r7).

3. *Report of the sixtieth session of the WHO Regional Committee for Europe.* Copenhagen, WHO Regional Office for Europe, 2010 (http://www.euro.who.int/en/who-we-are/governance/regional-committee-for-europe/past-sessions/sixtieth-session/documentation/report-of-the-sixtieth-session2).

4. *Report of the sixty-first session of the WHO Regional Committee for Europe.* Copenhagen, WHO Regional Office for Europe, 2011 (http://www.euro.who.int/en/who-we-are/governance/regional-committee-for-europe/sixty-first-session/documentation/report-of-the-sixty-first-session-of-the-who-regional-committee-for-europe).

5. *The new European policy for health – Health 2020: vision, values, main directions and approaches.* Copenhagen, WHO Regional Office for Europe, 2011 (EUR/RC61/9; http://www.euro.who.int/en/who-we-are/governance/regional-committee-for-europe/sixty-first-session/documentation/working-documents/wd9-the-new-european-policy-for-health-health-2020).

6. Health 2020 [web site]. Copenhagen, WHO Regional Office for Europe, 2011 (http://www.euro.who.int/en/what-we-do/event/first-meeting-of-the-european-health-policy-forum/health-2020).

7. *Interim first report on social determinants of health and the health divide in the WHO European Region.* Copenhagen, WHO Regional Office for Europe, 2010 (http://www.euro.who.int/en/what-we-do/health-topics/noncommunicable-diseases/obesity/publications/2010/interim-first-report-on-social-determinants-of-health-and-the-health-divide-in-the-who-european-region).

8. *Interim second report on social determinants of health and the health divide in the WHO European Region.* Copenhagen, WHO Regional Office for Europe, 2011 (EUR/RC61/Inf.Doc./5; http://www.euro.who.int/en/who-we-are/governance/regional-committee-for-europe/sixty-first-session/documentation/information-documents/inf-doc-5-the-health-divide-european-experiences-in-addressing-social-determinants-for-health).

[2] All electronic references were accessed on 20 June 2012.

9. *Governance for health in the 21st century.* Copenhagen, WHO Regional Office for Europe, 2011 (EUR/RC61/Inf.Doc./6; http://www.euro.who.int/en/who-we-are/governance/regional-committee-for-europe/sixty-first-session/documentation/information-documents/inf-doc-6-governance-of-health-in-the-21st-century).

10. *Strengthening public health capacities and services in Europe: a framework for action.* Copenhagen, WHO Regional Office for Europe, 2011 (EUR/RC61/10; http://www.euro.who.int/en/who-we-are/governance/regional-committee-for-europe/sixty-first-session/documentation/working-documents/wd10-strengthening-public-health-capacities-and-services-in-europe-a-framework-for-action).

11. *Action Plan for Implementation of the European Strategy for the Prevention and Control of Noncommunicable Diseases 2012–2016.* Copenhagen, WHO Regional Office for Europe, 2011 (EUR/RC61/12; http://www.euro.who.int/en/who-we-are/governance/regional-committee-for-europe/sixty-first-session/documentation/working-documents/wd12-action-plan-for-implementation-of-the-european-strategy-for-the-prevention-and-control-of-noncommunicable-diseases-20122016).

12. *European action plan to reduce the harmful use of alcohol 2012–2020.* Copenhagen, WHO Regional Office for Europe, 2011 (EUR/RC61/13; http://www.euro.who.int/en/who-we-are/governance/regional-committee-for-europe/sixty-first-session/documentation/working-documents/wd13-european-action-plan-to-reduce-the-harmful-use-of-alcohol-20122020).

13. *European Action Plan for HIV/AIDS 2012–2015.* Copenhagen, WHO Regional Office for Europe, 2011 (http://www.euro.who.int/en/what-we-publish/abstracts/european-action-plan-for-hivaids-20122015).

14. *Consolidated Action Plan to Prevent and Combat Multidrug- and Extensively Drug-resistant Tuberculosis in the WHO European Region 2011–2015.* Copenhagen, WHO Regional Office for Europe, 2011 (EUR/RC61/15; http://www.euro.who.int/en/who-we-are/governance/regional-committee-for-europe/sixty-first-session/documentation/working-documents/wd15-consolidated-action-plan-to-prevent-and-combat-multidrug-and-extensively-drug-resistant-tuberculosis-in-the-who-european-region-20112015).

15. *European strategic action plan on antibiotic resistance.* Copenhagen, WHO Regional Office for Europe, 2011 (EUR/RC61/14; http://www.euro.who.int/en/who-we-are/governance/regional-committee-for-europe/sixty-first-session/documentation/working-documents/wd14-european-strategic-action-plan-on-antibiotic-resistance).

16. *Partnerships for health in the European Region.* Copenhagen, WHO Regional Office for Europe, 2010 (EUR/RC60/12 Add. 1; http://www.euro.who.int/en/who-we-are/governance/regional-committee-for-europe/past-sessions/sixtieth-session/documentation/working-documents/eurrc6012-add.-1).

17. Implementation roadmaps for EC–WHO/Europe collaboration [web site]. Copenhagen, WHO Regional Office for Europe, 2011, (http://www.euro.who.int/en/who-we-are/partners/other-partners/european-union-eu-and-its-institutions2/european-commission-ec-senior-officials-meeting-som-2011/implementation-roadmaps-for-ec-whoeurope-collaboration).

18. *A country strategy for the WHO Regional Office for Europe.* Copenhagen, WHO Regional Office for Europe, 2011 (EUR/RC61/17 Rev.1; http://www.euro.who.int/en/who-we-are/governance/regional-committee-for-europe/sixty-first-

session/documentation/working-documents/wd17-a-country-strategy-for-the-who-regional-office-for-europe).

19. *Strengthening the role of the Regional Office's geographically dispersed offices (GDOs): a renewed GDO strategy for Europe.* Copenhagen, WHO Regional Office for Europe, 2011 (EUR/RC61/18; http://www.euro.who.int/en/who-we-are/governance/regional-committee-for-europe/sixty-first-session/documentation/working-documents/wd18-strengthening-the-role-of-the-regional-offices-geographically-dispersed-offices-gdos-a-renewed-gdo-strategy-for-europe).

20. *WHO reform for a healthy future.* Copenhagen, WHO Regional Office for Europe, 2011 (EUR/RC61/WG/Report; http://www.euro.who.int/en/who-we-are/governance/regional-committee-for-europe/sixty-first-session/documentation/report-of-discussions-on-who-reform).

21. Jakab Z. Embarking on developing the new European health policy – Health 2020. *European Journal of Public Health*, 2011, 21(1):130–132 (http://eurpub.oxfordjournals.org/content/21/1/130.full?sid=45e68bae-e18d-4f9b-b757-6c5027f15936).

22. Health 2020 [web site]. Copenhagen, WHO Regional Office for Europe, 2011 (http://www.euro.who.int/en/what-we-do/event/first-meeting-of-the-european-health-policy-forum/health-2020).

23. *The new European policy for health – Health 2020.* Copenhagen, WHO Regional Office for Europe, 2011 (EUR/RC61/Inf.Doc./4; http://www.euro.who.int/en/who-we-are/governance/regional-committee-for-europe/sixty-first-session/documentation/information-documents/inf-doc-4-the-new-european-policy-for-health-health-2020).

24. Eighteenth Standing Committee of the Regional Committee (2010–2011) [web site]. Copenhagen, WHO Regional Office for Europe, 2011 (http://www.euro.who.int/en/who-we-are/governance/standing-committee/eighteenth-standing-committee).

25. Nineteenth Standing Committee of the Regional Committee for Europe (2011–2012) [web site]. Copenhagen, WHO Regional Office for Europe, 2012 (http://www.euro.who.int/en/who-we-are/governance/standing-committee/nineteenth-standing-committee).

26. *Setting targets for Health 2020.* Copenhagen, WHO Regional Office for Europe, 2011 (EUR/RC61/Inf.Doc./7; http://www.euro.who.int/en/who-we-are/governance/regional-committee-for-europe/sixty-first-session/documentation/information-documents/inf-doc-7-setting-targets-for-health-2020).

27. *European countries take up the Health 2020 challenge.* Copenhagen, WHO Regional Office for Europe, 2011 (http://www.euro.who.int/en/who-we-are/regional-director/news/news/2011/03/european-countries-take-up-the-health-2020-challenge).

28. *Tallinn Charter: "Health Systems for Health and Wealth".* Copenhagen, WHO Regional Office for Europe, 2008 (http://www.euro.who.int/__data/assets/pdf_file/0008/88613/E91438.pdf).

29. *Executive Board special session on WHO reform. Geneva, 1–3 November 2011.* Geneva, World Health Organization, 2011 (EBSS/2/2011/REC/1; http://apps.who.int/gb/ebwha/pdf_files/EBSS2/EBSS2_REC1-en.pdf).

30. *The Rome Office of the WHO European Centre for Environment and Health (1991–2011): 20 years of experience.* Copenhagen, WHO Regional Office for Europe, 2011 (EUR/RC61/Inf.Doc./11;

http://www.euro.who.int/en/who-we-are/governance/regional-committee-for-europe/sixty-first-session/documentation/information-documents/inf-doc-11-rome).

31. *Consolidation of WHO/Europe's environment and health programmes.* Copenhagen, WHO Regional Office for Europe, 2011 (EUR/RC61/Inf. Doc./12; http://www.euro.who.int/en/who-we-are/governance/regional-committee-for-europe/sixty-first-session/documentation/information-documents/inf-doc-12-bonn-and-cph).

32. *World Health Assembly resolution WHA63.10 on partnerships.* Geneva, World Health Organization, 2010 (http://apps.who.int/gb/ebwha/pdf_files/WHA63-REC1/WHA63_REC1-en.pdf).

33. *Governance issues related to the European Observatory on Health Systems and Policies.* Copenhagen, WHO Regional Office for Europe, 2011 (EUR/RC61/20; http://www.euro.who.int/en/who-we-are/governance/regional-committee-for-europe/sixty-first-session/documentation/working-documents/wd20-summary-of-the-european-action-plan-for-hivaids-20122015).

34. Third Health Ministers' Forum – Health in All Policies in South-eastern Europe: a Shared Goal and Responsibility [web site]. Copenhagen, WHO Regional Office for Europe, 2011 (http://www.euro.who.int/en/what-we-do/health-topics/Health-systems/public-health-services/activities/south-eastern-europe-health-network-seehn/third-health-ministers-forum-health-in-all-policies-in-south-eastern-europe-a-shared-goal-and-responsibility).

35. *Banja Luka Pledge.* Copenhagen, WHO Regional Office for Europe, 2011 (http://www.euro.who.int/en/what-we-do/health-topics/Health-systems/public-health-services/activities/south-eastern-europe-health-network-seehn/third-health-ministers-forum-health-in-all-policies-in-south-eastern-europe-a-shared-goal-and-responsibility/documentation/banja-luka-pledge).

36. European Health for All Database (HFA-DB) [web site]. Copenhagen, WHO Regional Office for Europe, 2012 (http://www.euro.who.int/en/what-we-do/data-and-evidence/databases/european-health-for-all-database-hfa-db2).

37. Press releases [web site]. Copenhagen, WHO Regional Office for Europe, 2011 (http://www.euro.who.int/en/what-we-publish/information-for-the-media).

38. European Immunization Week. Prevent. Protect. Immunize [web site]. Copenhagen, WHO Regional Office for Europe, 2011 (http://eiw.euro.who.int).

39. *The programme budget as a strategic tool for accountability.* Copenhagen, WHO Regional Office for Europe, 2011 (EUR/RC61/Inf. Doc./10; http://www.euro.who.int/en/who-we-are/governance/regional-committee-for-europe/sixty-first-session/documentation/information-documents/inf-doc-10-programme-budget-as-a-strategic-tool-for-accountability).

40. Technical programmes in the European Region [web site]. Copenhagen, WHO Regional Office for Europe, 2011 (http://www.euro.who.int/en/who-we-are/technical-programmes-in-the-european-region).

41. European Centre for Disease Prevention and Control, WHO Regional Office for Europe. *HIV/AIDS surveillance report 2010.* Stockholm, European Centre for Disease Prevention and Control, 2010 (http://www.euro.who.int/en/what-we-do/health-topics/communicable-diseases/hivaids/publications/2011/hivaids-surveillance-in-europe-2010).

References

42. *Global health sector strategy on HIV/AIDS 2011–2015.* Geneva, World Health Organization, 2011 (http://whqlibdoc.who.int/publications/2011/9789241501651_eng.pdf).

43. *Getting to zero: UNAIDS 2011–2015 strategy.* Geneva, Joint United Nations Programme on HIV/AIDS (UNAIDS), 2010 (http://www.unaids.org/en/media/unaids/contentassets/documents/unaidspublication/2010/JC2034_UNAIDS_Strategy_en.pdf).

44. *Combating HIV/AIDS in the European Union and neighbouring countries, 2009–2013.* Brussels, Commission of the European Communities, 2009 (COM(2009)569 final; http://ec.europa.eu/health/ph_threats/com/aids/docs/com2009_en.pdf).

45. *Political Declaration on HIV and AIDS: Intensifying Our Efforts to Eliminate HIV and AIDS.* New York, United Nations, 2011 (http://www.un.org/Docs/asp/ws.asp?m=A/RES/65/277).

46. European Centre for Disease Prevention and Control, WHO Regional Office for Europe. *Tuberculosis surveillance in Europe 2008.* Stockholm, European Centre for Disease Prevention and Control, 2010 (http://www.euro.who.int/__data/assets/pdf_file/0007/78856/E93600.pdf).

47. *The Global Plan to Stop TB 2011–2015.* Geneva, World Health Organization, 2010 (http://www.stoptb.org/assets/documents/global/plan/TB_GlobalPlanToStopTB2011-2015.pdf).

48. *62nd World Health Assembly adopts resolution on MDR-TB and XDR-TB.* Geneva, World Health Organization, 2009 (http://www.who.int/tb/features_archive/wha62_15_tb_resolution/en/index.html).

49. *Roadmap to prevent and combat drug-resistant tuberculosis.* Copenhagen, WHO Regional Office for Europe, 2011 (http://www.euro.who.int/en/what-we-publish/abstracts/roadmap-to-prevent-and-combat-drug-resistant-tuberculosis).

50. Green Light Committee for the WHO European Region (GLC/Europe) [web site]. Copenhagen, WHO Regional Office for Europe, 2011 (http://www.euro.who.int/en/what-we-do/health-topics/communicable-diseases/tuberculosis/activities/green-light-committee-for-the-who-european-region-glceurope).

51. Malaria. Elimination from the WHO European Region by 2015 [web site]. Copenhagen, WHO Regional Office for Europe, 2012 (http://www.euro.who.int/en/what-we-do/health-topics/communicable-diseases/malaria).

52. *Tashkent Declaration: "The Move from Malaria Control to Elimination".* Copenhagen, WHO Regional Office for Europe, 2005 (http://www.euro.who.int/__data/assets/pdf_file/0005/98753/E89355.pdf).

53. WHO epidemiological briefs [web site]. Copenhagen, WHO Regional Office for Europe, 2012 (http://www.euro.who.int/en/what-we-do/health-topics/disease-prevention/vaccines-and-immunization/publications/who-epidemiological-briefs).

54. *Polio kicked out of Europe: European Region to retain polio-free status, but constant vigilance is needed.* Copenhagen, WHO Regional Office for Europe, 2011 (http://www.euro.who.int/en/what-we-publish/information-for-the-media/sections/latest-press-releases/polio-kicked-out-of-europe-european-region-to-retain-polio-free-status,-but-constant-vigilance-is-needed).

55. Online Laboratory Data Management System [web site]. Copenhagen, WHO Regional Office for Europe, 2011 (http://ldms.euro.who.int/Account/LogOn?ReturnUrl=%2f).

56. *Eliminating measles and rubella: framework for the verification process in the WHO European Region.* Copenhagen, WHO Regional Office for Europe, 2012 (http://www.euro.who.int/en/what-we-do/health-topics/communicable-diseases/measles-and-rubella/publications/2012/eliminating-measles-and-rubella-framework-for-the-verification-process-in-the-who-european-region).

57. European Immunization Week 2011 [web site]. Copenhagen, WHO Regional Office for Europe, 2011 (http://www.euro.who.int/en/what-we-do/health-topics/disease-prevention/vaccines-and-immunization/european-immunization-week/european-immunization-week-20052010/european-immunization-week-2011).

58. EuroFlu.org [web site]. Copenhagen, WHO Regional Office for Europe, 2011 (http://www.euroflu.org/index.php).

59. *WHO Regional Office for Europe guidance for sentinel influenza surveillance in humans.* Copenhagen, WHO Regional Office for Europe, 2011 (http://www.euro.who.int/en/what-we-do/health-topics/communicable-diseases/influenza/publications/2009/who-regional-office-for-europe-guidance-for-sentinel-influenza-surveillance-in-humans).

60. *Key changes to pandemic plans by Member States of the WHO European Region based on lessons learnt from the 2009 pandemic.* Copenhagen, WHO Regional Office for Europe, 2012 (http://www.euro.who.int/en/what-we-do/health-topics/communicable-diseases/influenza/publications/2012/key-changes-to-pandemic-plans-by-member-states-of-the-who-european-region-based-on-lessons-learnt-from-the-2009-pandemic).

61. Martirosyan L et al., EuroFlu group. The community impact of the 2009 influenza pandemic in the WHO European Region: a comparison with historical seasonal data from 28 countries. *BMC Infectious Diseases,* 2012, 12:36 (http://www.biomedcentral.com/1471-2334/12/36).

62. *Recommendations for good practice in pandemic preparedness: identified through evaluation of the response to pandemic (H1N1) 2009.* Copenhagen, WHO Regional Office for Europe, 2010 (http://www.euro.who.int/__data/assets/pdf_file/0017/128060/e94534.pdf).

63. *Final report of the IHR Review Committee published.* Copenhagen, WHO Regional Office for Europe, 2011 (http://www.euro.who.int/en/what-we-do/health-topics/communicable-diseases/influenza/news/news/2011/05/final-report-of-the-ihr-review-committee-published).

64. Pandemic Influenza Preparedness (PIP) Framework [web site]. Geneva, World Health Organization, 2012 (http://www.who.int/influenza/pip/en).

65. Influenza. Clinical management [web site]. Copenhagen, WHO Regional Office for Europe, 2012 (http://www.euro.who.int/en/what-we-do/health-topics/communicable-diseases/influenza/clinical-management).

66. World Health Day 2011 – Antibiotic resistance: No action today, no cure tomorrow [web site]. Copenhagen, WHO Regional Office for Europe, 2011 (http://www.euro.who.int/en/who-we-are/whd/past-themes-of-world-health-day/world-health-day-2011-antibiotic-resistance-no-action-today,-no-cure-tomorrow).

67. *Tackling antibiotic resistance from a food safety perspective in Europe*. Copenhagen, WHO Regional Office for Europe, 2011 (http://www.euro.who.int/__data/assets/pdf_file/0005/136454/e94889.pdf).

68. *Summary report on the regional high-level consultation on noncommunicable diseases (NCDs)*. Copenhagen, WHO Regional Office for Europe, 2011 (http://www.euro.who.int/en/what-we-do/event/regional-high-level-consultation-on-noncommunicable-diseases/summary-report-on-the-regional-high-level-consultation-on-noncommunicable-diseases-ncds).

69. *Political Declaration of the High-level Meeting of the General Assembly on the Prevention and Control of Non-communicable Diseases*. New York, United Nations, 2011 (http://www.un.org/Docs/asp/ws.asp?m=A/RES/66/2).

70. *Gaining health. The European strategy for the prevention and control of noncommunicable diseases*. Copenhagen, WHO Regional Office for Europe, 2006 (http://www.euro.who.int/__data/assets/pdf_file/0008/76526/E89306.pdf).

71. *Global strategy to reduce harmful use of alcohol*. Geneva, World Health Organization, 2010 (http://www.who.int/entity/substance_abuse/msbalcstragegy.pdf).

72. *European status report on alcohol and health 2010*. Copenhagen, WHO Regional Office for Europe, 2011 (http://www.euro.who.int/en/what-we-do/health-topics/disease-prevention/alcohol-use/publications/2010/european-status-report-on-alcohol-and-health-2010).

73. WHO FCTC. Framework Convention on Tobacco Control [web site]. Geneva, World Health Organization, 2012 (http://www.who.int/fctc/en/index.html).

74. *Empower women – Combating tobacco industry marketing in the WHO European Region*. Copenhagen, WHO Regional Office for Europe, 2010 (http://www.euro.who.int/en/what-we-do/health-topics/disease-prevention/tobacco/publications/2010/empower-women-combating-tobacco-industry-marketing-in-the-who-european-region).

75. World No Tobacco Day 2011: WHO Framework Convention on Tobacco Control [web site]. Copenhagen, WHO Regional Office for Europe 2011 (http://www.euro.who.int/en/what-we-do/health-topics/disease-prevention/tobacco/world-no-tobacco-day/2011-who-framework-convention-on-tobacco-control).

76. *European Childhood Obesity Surveillance Initiative (COSI)*. Copenhagen, WHO Regional Office for Europe, 2012 (http://www.euro.who.int/en/what-we-do/health-topics/disease-prevention/nutrition/policy/member-states-action-networks/childhood-obesity-surveillance/european-childhood-obesity-surveillance-initiative-cosi).

77. *WHO European database on nutrition, obesity and physical activity (NOPA)* [online database]. Copenhagen, WHO Regional Office for Europe, 2011 (http://data2.euro.who.int/nopa).

78. *WHO European Action Plan for Food and Nutrition Policy 2007–2012*. Copenhagen, WHO Regional Office for Europe, 2008 (http://www.euro.who.int/en/what-we-do/health-topics/noncommunicable-diseases/obesity/publications/pre-2009/who-european-action-plan-for-food-and-nutrition-policy-2007-2012).

79. *European Declaration on the Health of Children and Young People with Intellectual Disabilities*. Copenhagen, WHO Regional Office for Europe, 2010 (http://www.euro.who.int/en/what-we-

do/health-topics/noncommunicable-diseases/mental-health/publications/2010/european-declaration-on-the-health-of-children-and-young-people-with-intellectual-disabilities-and-their-families2).

80. *Mental health: facing the challenges, building solutions*. Copenhagen, WHO Regional Office for Europe, 2005 (http://www.euro.who.int/en/what-we-do/health-topics/noncommunicable-diseases/mental-health/publications/2005/mental-health-facing-the-challenges,-building-solutions).

81. Sethi D, Mitis F, Racioppi F. *Preventing injuries in Europe: from international collaboration to local implementation*. Copenhagen, WHO Regional Office for Europe, 2010 (http://www.euro.who.int/en/what-we-do/health-topics/disease-prevention/violence-and-injuries/publications/2010/preventing-injuries-in-europe-from-international-collaboration-to-local-implementation).

82. Sethi D et al., eds. *European report on preventing violence and knife crime among young people*. Copenhagen, WHO Regional Office for Europe, 2010 (http://www.euro.who.int/en/what-we-do/health-topics/disease-prevention/violence-and-injuries/publications/2010/european-report-on-preventing-violence-and-knife-crime-among-young-people).

83. Sethi D et al., eds. *European report on preventing elder maltreatment*. Copenhagen, WHO Regional Office for Europe, 2011 (http://www.euro.who.int/en/what-we-do/health-topics/disease-prevention/violence-and-injuries/publications/2011/european-report-on-preventing-elder-maltreatment).

84. Statistics and stories: improving the quality of maternal and neonatal health in Europe. *Entre Nous*, 2010, 70 (http://www.euro.who.int/en/what-we-do/health-topics/Life-stages/sexual-and-reproductive-health/publications/entre-nous/entre-nous/statistics-and-stories-improving-the-quality-of-maternal-and-neonatal-health-in-europe.-entre-nous-70,-2010).

85. Effective perinatal care training package (EPC) [web site]. Copenhagen, WHO Regional Office for Europe, 2012 (http://www.euro.who.int/en/what-we-do/health-topics/Life-stages/maternal-and-newborn-health/policy-and-tools/effective-perinatal-care-training-package-epc).

86. *Six success stories in Making Pregnancy Safer*. Copenhagen, WHO Regional Office for Europe, 2010 (http://www.euro.who.int/en/what-we-do/health-topics/Life-stages/maternal-and-newborn-health/publications/2010/six-success-stories-in-making-pregnancy-safer).

87. Improvement of maternal and child health in Kazakhstan. *Entre Nous*, 2011, 74 (http://www.euro.who.int/en/what-we-do/health-topics/Life-stages/maternal-and-newborn-health/publications/2011/improvement-of-maternal-and-child-health-in-kazakhstan,-entre-nous-74,-2011).

88. "Young people's health as a whole-of-society response" series [web site]. Copenhagen, WHO Regional Office for Europe, 2012 (http://www.euro.who.int/en/what-we-do/health-topics/Life-stages/sexual-and-reproductive-health/publications/2011/young-peoples-health-as-a-whole-of-society-response-series).

89. Currie C et al., eds. *Social determinants of health and well-being among young people. Health Behaviour in School-aged Children (HBSC) study: international report from the 2009/2010 survey*. Copenhagen, WHO Regional Office for Europe, 2012 (Health Policy for Children and Adolescents, No. 6; http://www.euro.who.int/en/what-we-publish/abstracts/social-determinants-

of-health-and-well-being-among-young-people.-health-behaviour-in-school-aged-children-hbsc-study).

90. *Improving hospital care for children. Case study report Armenia, Kazakhstan, Turkmenistan and Uzbekistan.* Copenhagen, WHO Regional Office for Europe, 2012 (http://www.euro.who.int/en/what-we-do/health-topics/Life-stages/child-and-adolescent-health/publications2/2010/improving-hospital-care-for-children.-case-study-report-armenia,-kazakhstan,-turkmenistan-and-uzbekistan).

91. WHO Regional Office for Europe, Federal Centre for Health Education (BZgA). *Standards for sexuality education in Europe. A framework for policy makers, educational and health authorities and specialists.* Cologne, BZgA, 2010 (http://www.bzga-whocc.de/pdf.php?id=061a863a0fdf28218e4fe9e1b3f463b3).

92. Entre Nous [web site]. Copenhagen, WHO Regional Office for Europe, 2012 (http://www.euro.who.int/en/what-we-do/health-topics/Life-stages/sexual-and-reproductive-health/publications/entre-nous/entre-nous).

93. *Progress regarding MDGs 3, 4 and 5. Draft conclusions from WHO meeting of national focal points for family and community health in Durres, Albania.* Copenhagen, WHO Regional Office for Europe, 2010 (http://www.euro.who.int/en/what-we-do/health-topics/Life-stages/maternal-and-newborn-health/news/news/2010/12/progress-regarding-mdgs-3,-4-and-5.-draft-conclusions-from-who-meeting-of-national-focal-points-for-family-and-community-health-in-durres,-albania.).

94. *Progress towards Millennium Development Goals 4, 5 and 6 in the WHO European Region: 2011 update.* Copenhagen, WHO Regional Office for Europe, 2011 (http://www.euro.who.int/en/what-we-do/health-topics/health-determinants/millenium-development-goals/publications2/2012/progress-towards-millennium-development-goals-4,-5-and-6-in-the-who-european-region-2011-update).

95. *Ottawa Charter for Health Promotion, 1986.* Copenhagen, WHO Regional Office for Europe, 1986 (http://www.euro.who.int/en/who-we-are/policy-documents/ottawa-charter-for-health-promotion,-1986).

96. *Summary interim report on implementation of the Tallinn Charter.* Copenhagen, WHO Regional Office for Europe, 2011 (EUR/RC61/11; http://www.euro.who.int/en/who-we-are/governance/regional-committee-for-europe/sixty-first-session/documentation/working-documents/wd11-summary-interim-report-on-implementation-of-the-tallinn-charter).

97. *Health systems for better health: the WHO/Europe package of support for health systems strengthening.* Copenhagen, WHO Regional Office for Europe, 2011 (EUR/RC61/Inf.Doc./9; http://www.euro.who.int/en/who-we-are/governance/regional-committee-for-europe/sixty-first-session/documentation/information-documents/inf-doc-9-health-systems-for-better-health-the-whoeurope-package-of-support-for-health-systems-strengthening).

98. Health financing policy papers series [web site]. Copenhagen, WHO Regional Office for Europe, 2010 (http://www.euro.who.int/en/what-we-do/health-topics/Health-systems/health-systems-financing/publications2/2010/health-financing-policy-papers-series).

99. *The world health report 2010. Health systems financing: the path to universal coverage.* Geneva, World Health Organization, 2010 (http://www.who.int/whr/2010/en/index.html).

100. European public health action plan [web site]. Copenhagen, WHO Regional Office for Europe, 2012 (http://www.euro.who.int/en/what-we-do/health-topics/Health-systems/public-health-services/policy/european-public-health-action-plan).

101. Towards a new European public health action plan. In: WHO/Europe public health forum [web site]. Copenhagen, WHO Regional Office for Europe, 2012 (http://discussion.euro.who.int/forum/topics/towards-a-new-european-public-health-action-plan).

102. *WHO Global Code of Practice on the International Recruitment of Health Personnel*. Geneva, World Health Organization, 2010 (http://www.who.int/entity/hrh/migration/code/code_en.pdf).

103. *Patients' safety: 2nd round table on reporting systems in health care*. Copenhagen, WHO Regional Office for Europe, 2012 (http://www.euro.who.int/en/what-we-do/health-topics/Health-systems/patient-safety/publications2/2012/patients-safety-2nd-round-table-on-reporting-systems-in-health-care).

104. Health Systems in Transition (HiT) series [web site]. Copenhagen, European Observatory on Health Systems and Policies, 2012 (http://www.euro.who.int/en/who-we-are/partners/observatory/health-system-reviews-hits/full-list-of-hits).

105. Wismar M et al., eds. *Cross-border health care in the European Union. Mapping and analysing practices and policies*. Copenhagen, WHO Regional Office for Europe, 2011 (Observatory Studies Series, No. 22; http://www.euro.who.int/en/who-we-are/partners/observatory/studies/cross-border-health-care-in-the-european-union.-mapping-and-analysing-practices-and-policies).

106. *Protecting children's health in a changing environment. Report of the Fifth Ministerial Conference on Environment and Health*. Copenhagen, WHO Regional Office for Europe, 2010 (http://www.euro.who.int/en/what-we-publish/abstracts/protecting-childrens-health-in-a-changing-environment.-report-of-the-fifth-ministerial-conference-on-environment-and-health).

107. *Report of the first session of the European Environment and Health Task Force*. Copenhagen, WHO Regional Office for Europe, 2011 (http://www.euro.who.int/en/what-we-do/health-topics/environment-and-health/european-process-on-environment-and-health/governance/european-environment-and-health-task-force-ehtf/report-of-the-first-session-of-the-european-environment-and-health-task-force).

108. Environment and Health Information System (ENHIS) [web site]. Copenhagen, WHO Regional Office for Europe, 2012 (http://www.euro.who.int/en/what-we-do/data-and-evidence/environment-and-health-information-system-enhis).

109. *WHO guidelines for indoor air quality: selected pollutants*. Copenhagen, WHO Regional Office for Europe, 2010 (http://www.euro.who.int/__data/assets/pdf_file/0009/128169/e94535.pdf).

110. *Burden of disease from environmental noise. Quantification of healthy life years lost in Europe*. Copenhagen, WHO Regional Office for Europe, 2011 (http://www.euro.who.int/__data/assets/pdf_file/0008/136466/e94888.pdf).

111. *Environmental burden of disease associated with inadequate housing. Summary report*. Copenhagen, WHO Regional Office for Europe, 2011 (http://www.euro.who.int/en/what-we-do/health-topics/environment-and-health/Housing-and-health/

publications/2011/environmental-burden-of-disease-associated-with-inadequate-housing.-summary-report).

112. *Small scale water supplies in the pan-European Region. Background. Challenges. Improvements.* Copenhagen, WHO Regional Office for Europe, 2011 (http://www.euro.who.int/__data/assets/pdf_file/0018/140355/e94968.pdf).

113. Health economic assessment tool (HEAT) for cycling and walking [web site]. Copenhagen, WHO Regional Office for Europe, 2011 (http://www.euro.who.int/en/what-we-do/health-topics/environment-and-health/Transport-and-health/activities/promotion-of-safe-walking-and-cycling-in-urban-areas/quantifying-the-positive-health-effects-of-cycling-and-walking/health-economic-assessment-tool-heat-for-cycling-and-walking).

114. *Sources and effects of ionizing radiation. United Nations Scientific Committee on the Effects of Atomic Radiation. UNSCEAR 2008 Report to the General Assembly with Scientific Annexes. Annex D. Health effects due to radiation from the Chernobyl accident.* New York, United Nations, 2011 (http://www.unscear.org/docs/reports/2008/11-80076_Report_2008_Annex_D.pdf).

115. International Health Regulations (IHR) [web site]. Geneva, World Health Organization, 2012 (http://www.who.int/ihr/about/en/index.html).

116. International Health Regulations. Past meetings [web site]. Copenhagen, WHO Regional Office for Europe, 2011 (http://www.euro.who.int/en/what-we-do/health-topics/emergencies/international-health-regulations/activities/past-meetings).

117. *Assessment of health systems' crisis preparedness: Turkey*. Copenhagen, WHO Regional Office for Europe, 2010 (http://www.euro.who.int/en/what-we-do/health-topics/emergencies/disaster-preparedness-and-response/publications/2011/assessment-of-health-systems-crisis-preparedness-turkey).

118. *Strengthening health-system emergency preparedness. Toolkit for assessing health-system capacity for crisis management. Part 1. User manual.* Copenhagen, WHO Regional Office for Europe, 2012 (http://www.euro.who.int/en/what-we-do/health-topics/emergencies/disaster-preparedness-and-response/publications/2012/strengthening-health-system-emergency-preparedness.-toolkit-for-assessing-health-system-capacity-for-crisis-management.-part-1.-user-manual).

119. *Hospital emergency response checklist*. Copenhagen, WHO Regional Office for Europe, 2011 (http://www.euro.who.int/en/what-we-do/health-topics/emergencies/disaster-preparedness-and-response/publications/2011/hospital-emergency-response-checklist).

120. *Health advice for travellers to 2012 UEFA football championship*. Copenhagen, WHO Regional Office for Europe, 2012 (http://www.euro.who.int/en/what-we-do/health-topics/emergencies/disaster-preparedness-and-response/publications/2012/health-advice-for-travellers-to-2012-uefa-football-championship).

121. *The WHO e-atlas of disaster risk for the European Region. Volume 1. Exposure to natural hazards. Version 2.0*. Copenhagen, WHO Regional Office for Europe, 2011 (http://www.euro.who.int/en/what-we-publish/abstracts/who-e-atlas-of-disaster-risk-for-the-european-region-the.-volume-1.-exposure-to-natural-hazards.-version-2.0).

122. Outbreaks of *E. coli* O104:H4 infection [web site]. Copenhagen, WHO Regional Office for Europe, 2011 (http://www.euro.who.int/en/what-we-do/health-topics/emergencies/international-health-regulations/outbreaks-of-e.-coli-o104h4-infection).

123. Interactive atlases [web site]. Copenhagen, WHO Regional Office for Europe, 2012 (http://www.euro.who.int/en/what-we-do/data-and-evidence/equity-in-health/interactive-atlases).

124. Web-based resource of examples of health system action on socially determined health inequalities [web site]. Copenhagen, WHO Regional Office for Europe, 2012 (http://www.euro.who.int/en/what-we-do/data-and-evidence/equity-in-health/web-based-resource).

125. *Putting our own house in order: examples of health-system action on socially determined health inequalities.* Copenhagen, WHO Regional Office for Europe, 2010 (Studies on social and economic determinants of population health, No. 5; http://www.euro.who.int/en/what-we-publish/abstracts/putting-our-own-house-in-order-examples-of-health-system-action-on-socially-determined-health-inequalities).

126. Joint policy briefs and policy summaries [web site]. Copenhagen, WHO Regional Office for Europe, 2012 (http://www.euro.who.int/en/what-we-do/data-and-evidence/health-evidence-network-hen/publications/joint-policy-briefs-and-policy-summaries).

127. Mossialos E et al. *Policies and incentives for promoting innovation in antibiotic research.* Copenhagen, WHO Regional Office for Europe, 2010 (http://www.euro.who.int/en/who-we-are/partners/observatory/studies/policies-and-incentives-for-promoting-innovation-in-antibiotic-research).

128. Kutzin J, Cashin C, Jakab M. *Implementing health financing reform: lessons from countries in transition.* Copenhagen, WHO Regional Office for Europe, 2010 (Observatory Studies Series, No. 21; http://www.euro.who.int/en/who-we-are/partners/observatory/studies/implementing-health-financing-reform-lessons-from-countries-in-transition).

129. Saltman RB, Durán A, Dubois HFW. *Governing public hospitals. Reform strategies and the movement towards institutional autonomy.* Copenhagen, WHO Regional Office for Europe, 2011 (Observatory Studies Series, No. 25; http://www.euro.who.int/en/what-we-publish/abstracts/governing-public-hospitals.-reform-strategies-and-the-movement-towards-institutional-autonomy).

130. Figueras J, McKee M, eds. *Health systems, health, wealth and societal well-being. Assessing the case for investing in health systems.* Maidenhead, Open University Press, 2011 (European Observatory on Health Systems and Policies series; http://www.euro.who.int/en/who-we-are/partners/observatory/studies/health-systems,-health,-wealth-and-societal-well-being.-assessing-the-case-for-investing-in-health-systems).

ANNEX.
IMPLEMENTATION OF THE PROGRAMME BUDGET FOR 2010–2011

The assessment process for the programme budget evaluates the Secretariat's contribution to the achievement of the Organization-wide expected results (OWERS) and performance indicators according to each of WHO's 13 strategic objectives (SOs). As a measure for improving its performance, the assessment is an integral part of WHO's results-based management and commitment to accountability in the use of resources. This assessment coincides with the comprehensive programmatic, managerial and administrative reform of WHO, so it provides lessons that can inform the reform process. This process in turn lays a foundation for the new Twelfth General Programme of Work, a strategic framework for the work of WHO for 2014–2020.

Achievement of the OWERs is assessed primarily by the achievement of indicators. In this assessment, the baseline and target values were adjusted to reflect assessment of the implementation of the programme budget for 2008–2009. Some baselines and targets were updated to reflect further clarification of the definitions and measurement criteria for individual indicators. The assessment of the OWERS is a bottom-up self-assessment, in which individual offices, from country to regional level, review their performance in achieving office-specific expected results (OSERs) through delivering planned products and services. The assessment identifies achievements, success factors, constraints and lessons learnt.

Overview of technical implementation

Table 1 and Fig. 1 give an overview of attainment of the OWERs and Table 2 and Fig. 2 summarize the attainment of the OSERs by SO. They show that 12 of the 85 OWERs were assessed as partly or not achieved[1] and 8% of OSERs were assessed as at risk or in trouble. This was primarily due to shortage of funding, including cases when this led to a shortage of technical staff to support delivery. Other persistent implementation challenges in the WHO Regional Office for Europe include delays in recruitment processes, excessively specified voluntary contributions, late release of funds and the limitations of the Global Management System, leading to insufficient monitoring.

Resources and their implementation

Tables 3 and 4 and Fig. 3 and 4 show how the Regional Office's programme budget for 2010–2011 was financed and implemented, by budget segment and SO.

In WHO globally, the 2010–2011 biennium presented a challenge in the form of lower-than-expected voluntary contributions, especially in the base-programmes segment of the budget. This meant that some areas were not as well financed as had been planned, and were therefore unable to achieve their target implementation. Although

[1] An OWER is fully achieved when all indicator targets are met or surpassed, partly achieved when one or more indicator targets are not met and not achieved when no indicator targets are met.

TABLE 1. Achievement of OWERs by SO, WHO Regional Office for Europe, 2010–2011

SO	Content	OWERs			
		Fully achieved	Partly achieved	Not achieved	Total
1	Communicable diseases	7	1	1	9
2	HIV/AIDS, tuberculosis and malaria	6	0	0	6
3	Chronic noncommunicable conditions	5	1	0	6
4	Child, adolescent, maternal, sexual and reproductive health and ageing	8	0	0	8
5	Emergencies and disasters	6	1	0	7
6	Risk factors for health	6	0	0	6
7	Social and economic determinants of health	3	2	0	5
8	Healthier environment	6	0	0	6
9	Nutrition and food safety	6	0	0	6
10	Health systems and services	10	2	1	13
11	Medical products and technologies	3	0	0	3
12	WHO leadership, governance and partnerships	4	0	0	4
13	Enabling and support functions	3	3	0	6
Total		**73**	**10**	**2**	**85**

FIG. 1. Achievement of OWERs by SO, WHO Regional Office for Europe, 2010–2011

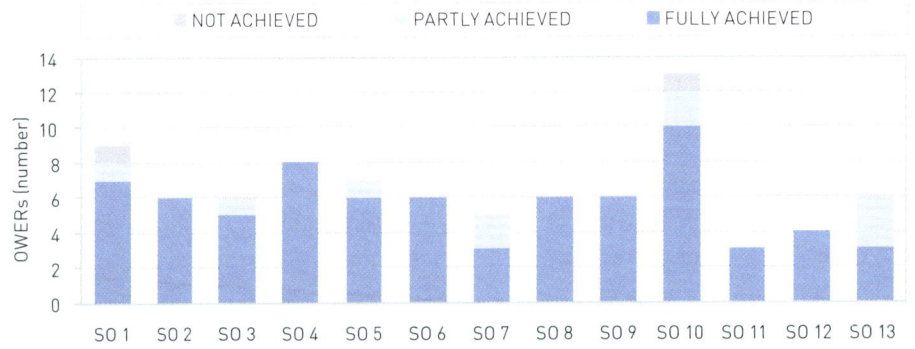

Annex. Implementation of the programme budget for 2010–2011

TABLE 2. Achievement of OSERs by SO, WHO Regional Office for Europe, 2010–2011

SO	Content	OSERs (number)	OSERs (%)		OSERs (%)		
			Reported	Not reported	On track	At risk	In trouble
1	Communicable diseases	125	72	28	93	7	0
2	HIV/AIDS, tuberculosis and malaria	51	84	16	95	2	2
3	Chronic noncommunicable conditions	81	98	2	91	9	0
4	Child, adolescent, maternal, sexual and reproductive health, and ageing	40	100	0	98	0	3
5	Emergencies and disasters	72	99	1	94	4	1
6	Risk factors for health	62	94	6	91	7	2
7	Social and economic determinants of health	31	100	0	77	10	13
8	Healthier environment	59	80	20	79	6	15
9	Nutrition and food safety	31	81	19	88	4	8
10	Health systems and services	136	99	1	86	9	5
11	Medical products and technologies	53	98	2	90	4	6
12	WHO leadership, governance and partnerships	100	90	10	91	2	7
13	Enabling and support functions	203	94	6	99	1	0
Total		1044	91	9	92	5	3

FIG. 2. Achievement of OSERs by SO, WHO Regional Office for Europe, 2010–2011

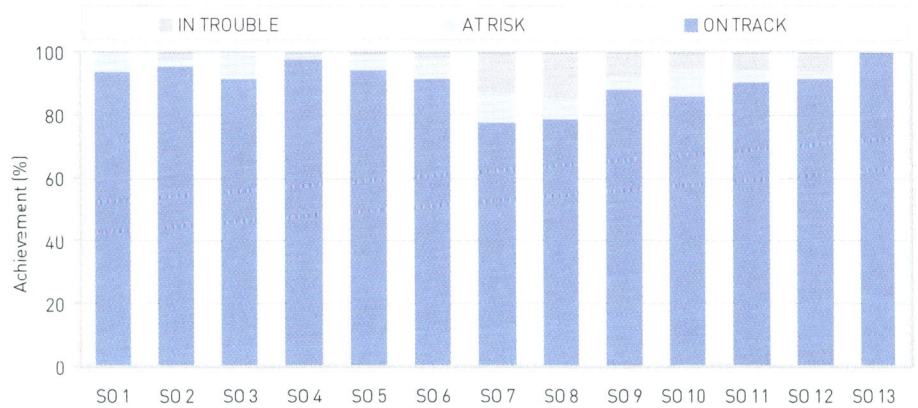

82% of the base-programmes segment in the Regional Office was funded (the highest level among the WHO regions), SOs 1, 4, 5, 10 and 11 had less than 70% of planned funding, and thus less than 60% implementation of the approved budget. Technical SOs 10 and 11 showed the lowest levels of available funds (58% and 52%, respectively).

Overall US$ 209 million (or 91% of available funds) was spent on implementing activities.

This high level of funding and implementation meant a high level of results, but also reduced the carry-forward compared to the 2008–2009 biennium; that is, implementation exceeded the new income received. SOs 4–6, 10 and 11 had the highest implementation rates of available funds (all above 90%), almost completely exhausting their available resources. These SOs thus started the new biennium relying almost entirely on new funds to be received.

TABLE 3. Programme budget for 2010–2011 (US$ millions), financial implementation by segments, WHO Regional Office for Europe

Segment	Funds		Funds available as % of approved budget	Implementation as of 31 December 2011	Implementation as % of:	
	Approved budget	Available as of 31 December 2011			approved budget	funds available
Base programmes	239	196	82	180	75	92
Special programmes and collaborative arrangements	15	27	181	23	157	87
Outbreak and crisis response	8	6	74	5	67	91
Total	**262**	**229**	**87**	**209**	**80**	**91**

FIG. 3. Programme budget for 2010–2011, financial implementation by segments, WHO Regional Office for Europe

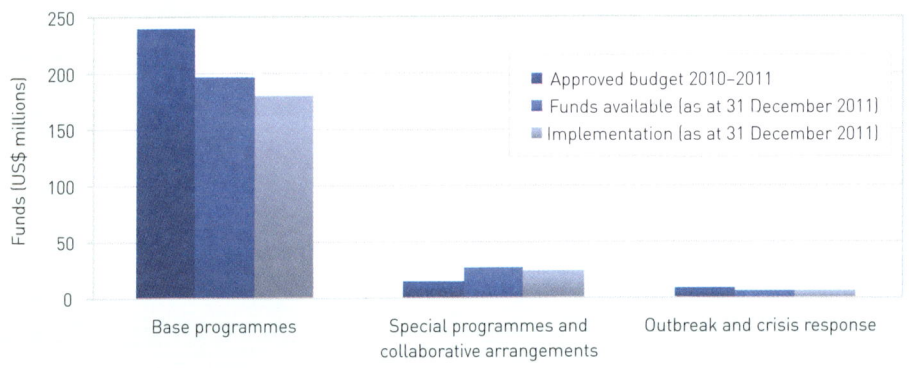

Annex. Implementation of the programme budget for 2010–2011

During 2010–2011, several adjustments were made to harmonize the planning of expenditure on SOs 12 and 13, resulting in an artificial underimplementation of the programme budget for SO 13 and overimplementation for SO 12.

Taken together, the parts of the programme budget devoted to these two SOs were fully implemented.

The special programmes and collaborative arrangements were financed above the level of

TABLE 4. Programme budget for 2010–2011 (US$ millions), financial implementation by SO, base programmes, WHO Regional Office for Europe

SO	Funds		Funds available as % of approved budget	Implementation as of 31 December 2011	Implementation as % of:	
	Approved budget	Available as of 31 December 2011			approved budget	funds available
1	23	15	65	12	53	82
2	30	23	76	20	68	89
3	15	13	86	11	72	84
4	13	8	62	8	58	95
5	11	7	63	6	57	91
6	10	9	88	8	82	93
7	7	7	100	6	88	88
8	17	19	108	16	93	86
9	6	6	108	5	93	86
10	41	24	58	22	54	93
11	6	3	52	3	47	90
12	26	31	123	31	121	99
13	37	33	91	33	89	98
Total	239	196	82	180	75	92

FIG. 4. Programme budget for 2010–2011, financial implementation by SO, base programmes, WHO Regional Office for Europe

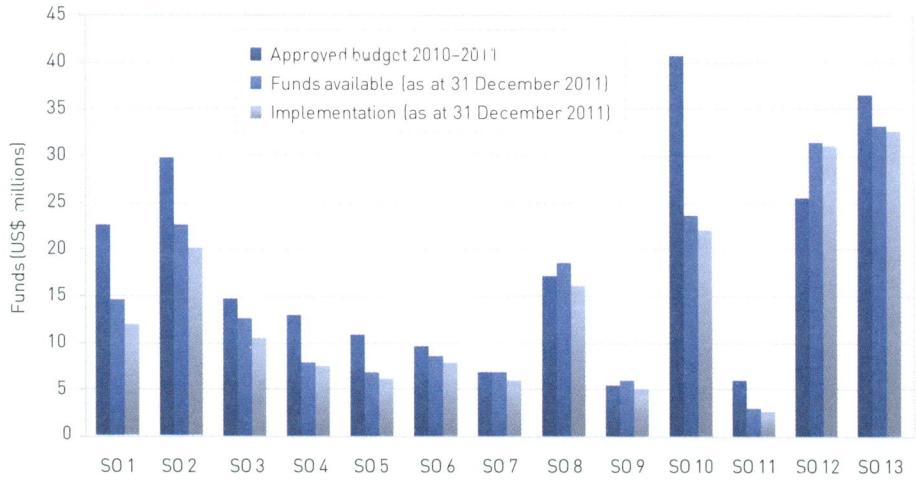

the approved programme budget, requiring some shifts in the programme-budget level during the biennium. The available resources of this budget segment were implemented at 87%.

Outbreak and crisis response was financed at 74% of the approved budget, with 91% of funds being implemented during the biennium.

In the 2010–2011 biennium, the Regional Office paid extra attention to performance assessment. In 2010, the WHO Regional Committee for Europe endorsed changes to its governance functions and methods of work, and those of the Standing Committee of the Regional Committee (SCRC). One of the changes gave the SCRC an oversight role in assessing performance and accountability. The Secretariat therefore regularly presented the SCRC with standardized management reports and narrative analytical reports, with key data on technical programmes' implementation status and summaries of outputs and deliverables.

Moreover, as a response to the Regional Committee's request for a tool to strengthen its governance and oversight functions, the Secretariat, working with members of the Eighteenth SCRC, prepared a strategic tool for increased accountability, enhanced management of resources and improved quality of funding. It will be pilot-tested during the 2012–2013 biennium within the context of the WHO reform process.